Complications in
Male Circumcision

Complications in Male Circumcision

Edited by

MOHAMED A BAKY FAHMY, MD, FRCS
Professor
Pediatric Surgery
Al Azher University
Cairo, Egypt

ELSEVIER

Publisher: Cathleen Sether
Acquisition Editor: Belinda Kuhn
Editorial Project Manager: Rebeka Henry
Production Project Manager: Sreejith Viswanathan
Cover Designer: Christian Bilbow

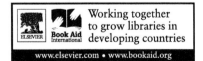

Working together
to grow libraries in
developing countries

www.elsevier.com • www.bookaid.org

List of Contributors

Ahmad R. Abdel-Aal, MS
Role of Hyperbaric Oxygen Therapy in MC
    Complications
Surgery Department
Assuit University
Assuit, Egypt

Jonathan A. Allan, PhD
Canada Research Chair in Queer Theory
Faculty of Arts
Brandon University
Brandon, Manitoba, Canada

Anthony Emmanuel, BSc (Hons), DipRD, MD (Res), MRCS (Eng)
Urology Registrar
Solihull Hospital
Solihull, United Kingdom

Mohamed A Baky Fahmy, MD, FRCS
Professor
Pediatric Surgery
Al Azher University
Cairo, Egypt

Atieno Kili K'Odhiambo, PhD
Senior Lecturer
Department of Educational Foundations
University of Nairobi
Nairobi, Kenya

Nick Watkin, MA, MChir, FRCS (Urol)
Consultant Urologist and Professor in Urology
St George's University Hospitals
London, United Kingdom

Preface

Circumcision remains as one of the most controversial topics in current medical practice. The most important argument against circumcision is the permanent change of anatomy, histology and function of the penis, with potential complications, which were reported to be low in developed countries, whereas the rate of complication may be up to 45% when circumcision is carried out by traditional circumcisers rather than by medically trained professionals in developing countries. In some studies reporting the complications of circumcision, primary haemorrhage was the most common (52%) complication, whereas infection, meatal stenosis, incomplete circumcision, penile oedema, glanular injury, penile adhesions, iatrogenic hypospadias and urethral injuries were also detected at different rates.

There are minor complications after circumcision that cannot be avoided even when the procedure is undertaken by specialized paediatric surgeons or urologists in properly equipped centres, especially if the child or his penis is congenitally abnormal, for example, circumcising a child with excessive suprapubic fat or a child with webbed penis or microphallus.

After practicing circumcision and managing other surgeons complications in thousands of boys for 35 years in a country like Egypt (with about 90% circumcision rate), I found parents had a great urge to do this surgery even for a handicapped or critically ill child, with a possibility for higher rate of complications. So the best way to minimize complications of male circumcision (MC) and to compete against its serious effects on male health is to standardize the MC procedure and to educate both families and physicians about the potential complications and how they could manage it early and promptly.

The spectrum of post-MC complications is so wide to be discussed, so we will just focus on both the common and the uncommon complications that usually raise a debate about their management. There are different ways to classify MC complications: early or late, minor or major, local or systemic and rare or common.

PHOTO CREDITS

I'm so grateful to all my colleagues who allowed me to use some of their photos and to the parents who consented me to use the photos of their children for demonstration.

Abbreviations and Acronyms

AAP	American Academy of Pediatrics
AIDS	Acquired immunodeficiency syndrome
ALAT	Alanine aminotransferase
BXO	Balanitis xerotica obliterans
CDC	Centers for Disease Control and Prevention
CI	Confidence interval
EMLA	Eutectic Mixture of Local Anaesthetics
HBO	Hyperbaric oxygen
HBV	Hepatitis B virus
HCV	Hepatitis C virus
HIV	Human immunodeficiency virus
HPV	Human papilloma virus
MC	Male circumcision
NIS	Nationwide Inpatient Sample
STI	Sexually transmitted infection
UNAIDS	Joint United Nations Programme on HIV/AIDS
VMMC	Voluntary medical male circumcision
WHO	World Health Organization

Contents

CHAPTER 1

Introduction

MOHAMED A BAKY FAHMY, MD, FRCS

Male circumcision (MC) is usually practised for religious, social, cultural and medical reasons. It is one of the oldest and most common surgical procedures performed globally. It is estimated that one-third of men worldwide are circumcised, two-thirds of whom are Muslims. The procedure is most commonly practised in the Muslim world, Israel (where it is near-universal for religious reasons), the United States and parts of Southeast Asia and Africa. It is relatively rare in Europe, Latin America, parts of Southern Africa and most of Asia. Circumcision is performed approximately 1.2 million times each year in the United States (Fig. 1.1).

Global MC prevalence was 38.7% (95% confidence interval [CI]: 33.4, 43.9). Approximately half of the circumcisions were for religious and cultural reasons. For countries lacking data, such as Egypt, it is assumed that at least 90% of Muslims are circumcised. The most common procedure for children in US hospitals is prophylactic vaccination (1,329,600) followed by MC (1,147,700), making MC the most common procedure in boys. With 15 million circumcisions per year, each taking about 20 min, it means that approximately 500 men are being circumcised right now.

Neonatal circumcision rates are declining across several countries including Canada and most of the European countries, and this may be a reflection of changing demographic patterns and parental beliefs occasioned by studies in psychology, especially Freudian psychoanalytic theory, which maintains that the trauma inflicted on neonates lasts for life. The human rights movements might have also altered the thinking of many parents. The Centers for Disease Control and Prevention (CDC) report showed a decreasing trend in US circumcision rates from 1999 to 2000 until 2008–2010 from 60% to 55% of newborn males. In the United Kingdom, between 1997 and 2004, circumcision rates declined from 2.6/1000 boys/year to 2.1/1000 boys/year.

It is almost unbelievable that removal or nonremoval of this small piece of skin from the head of the penis has actually been the focus of medical and social attention

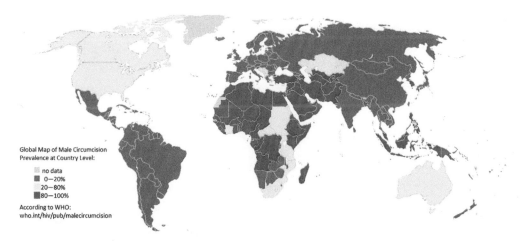

FIG. 1.1 Global map of male circumcision prevalence by country, according to the sources from the Circumcision Reference and Commentary Service (https://www.who.int/hiv/pub/malecircumcision/infopack_en_2.pdf - 651k).

Complications in Male Circumcision. https://doi.org/10.1016/B978-0-323-68127-8.00001-6

and debate for hundreds of years A Google search for 'circumcision' produces about 11 million results in 0.58 seconds and a PubMed search for 'male circumcision' shows 7631 published articles.

The spectrum of post-MC complications is so wide, and there are different ways to classify these complications: early or late, minor or major, local or systemic and rare or common.

Recently, I realized that these complications could be due to either a practitioner's fault or family malpractice, as most parents had a great urge to do this surgery even for a handicapped or critically ill child; as you can see the child in Fig. 1.2 who had a hip spica cast for bilateral hip dislocations, but his family insisted to do circumcision for him. At the same time, a mother's lacking of knowledges and negligence in dealing with a circumcised baby may complicate a properly done procedure.

During the past three decades, most of the publications and debates have focussed mainly on either fighting against MC and trying to prove that it is a mutilation of the penis and should be abandoned by publishing articles about remote and nonrealistic complications, such as nightmares and body-loss grief, or endeavouring to prove the benefits and advantages of MC up to recommending it as a vaccine against sexually transmitted diseases through biased studies, in my opinion.

But awareness about MC complications is not widely discussed or elaborated impartially, and little attention is paid to implement the methods to avoid such complications and its impact on the child's future, especially in abnormal babies or in those with deformed penises.

So the best way, in my opinion, to minimize complications of MC and to compete against its serious effect on male health is to standardize the procedure, especially in communities that will continue to practice MC in a religious background, and to educate both families and physicians about the potential complications, how to avoid them and how to manage them early and properly.

The main importance of studying MC complications is that it helps justify the benefits of routine circumcision in newborns as a preventative health measure and to see how far the benefits exceed the risks of the procedure, or vice versa. The most important study in this regard was conducted in the United States, in which the complication rates of undergoing or not undergoing circumcision were studied. The study was performed on 136,000 boys born in army hospitals between 1980 and 1985. Among them, 100,000 were circumcised and 193 (0.19%) had complications, mostly minor, with no deaths, but of the 36,000 who were not circumcised the problems of urinary tract infection (UTI) and other diseases were more than 10 times higher and there were 2 deaths.[1] Another Nationwide Inpatient Sample (NIS) study done in the United States estimated a death rate of 1 per 49,166 circumcisions (with another comorbidity).[2] Such sort of studies should be implemented in other developing counties with a high rate of MC.

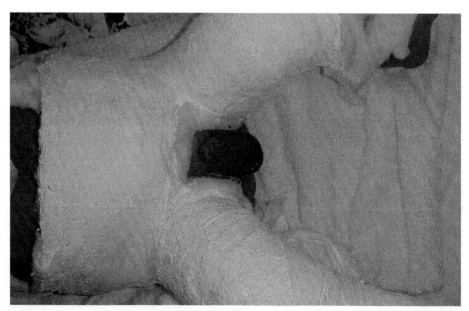

FIG. 1.2 A male newborn with bilateral femur fractures, but his parents insisted to have him circumcised.

DEFINITIONS

It is crucial to define precisely the meaning of complications, their spectrum and their effects because many respectable journals with a high impact factor and a high rate of citation may publish a study encountering unrelated MC complications, such as anaesthetic drug side effects, as complications of MC, and also many authors may resort to mangling the psychic problems of a certain group of people as a general complication of MC, as we can see in papers discussing self-esteem and sexual dissatisfaction. On the other side, many articles are trying to support MC by publishing false data about the role of circumcision in the prevention of many disorders, such as malignant diseases, not only in those who were circumcised but also in their female partners.

A major challenge in reviewing the published studies of MC complications is the standardization of the definition of complications; for example, many publications consider incomplete removal of the foreskin as a complication and as an adverse outcome that may involve further surgery, but it is not an actual medical complication per se. Also precise definitions are not often given for bleeding as a complication, which may be a minimal oozing readily stopped by compression or a more severe bleeding requiring a blood transfusion. Therefore to report complications as consistently as possible between studies, an agreement has to be achieved between scholars about the definition of complications of MC. The rate of complications is another misleading issue, as one case of complete penile loss following gangrene complicating MC among 10,000 cases is a serious and alarming problem and difficult to be counted as a low rate of complication (1/10,000).[3]

What Is Male Circumcision?

Circumcision is the surgical removal of the foreskin, the fold of skin that covers the head of the penis. It is widely practised for religious and traditional reasons, often within the first 2 weeks after birth, or at the beginning of adolescence as a rite of passage into adulthood. It may also be performed for medical reasons to treat problems involving the foreskin or the penis.

In Hebrew, circumcision is called peritomy, from the Greek *peritome*, but in Latin, *circumcisionem* (nominative *circumcisio*) is a noun of action from past participle stem of circumcidere 'to cut around; cut, clip, trim' (from *circum* 'around' and *caedere* 'to cut') signifies cutting and, specifically, removal of the prepuce, or foreskin, from the penis.

Generally, circumcision means cutting around an anatomic part, the surgical removal of a part or the entire prepuce; the term 'peritomy' is not commonly used.

Circumcision is known in Arabic as 'Al-Tohour', and it is also known as 'tahera', which means purification. It is known as 'tohara' in Kiswahili (the dominant language in East Africa), meaning cleansing accompanied with education, in the traditional sense. There is another name for circumcision in Arabic that is used only by religious scholars and has an impact on the definition of the procedure: 'Khitan', which means just cutting without any reference to purification or definition of how much to remove from the prepuce.

Definition of Complications

In most medical dictionaries, a complication is defined as an unanticipated problem that arises following, and is a result of, a procedure, treatment or illness. A complication is so named because it complicates the situation and makes it difficult to manage.

In Wikipedia, a medical complication is defined as an unfavourable evolution or consequence of a disease, a health condition or a therapy. The disease may become worse in its severity or show a higher number of signs, symptoms or new pathologic changes and become widespread throughout the body or affect other organ systems. A new disease may also appear as a complication to a previously existing one. Medical treatment, such as using drugs or surgery, may produce adverse effects or new health problem(s) by itself. Therefore a complication may be iatrogenic (i.e. literally brought forth by the physician). Disorders that are concomitant but are not caused by the other disorder are comorbidities.

The Dindo classification defines a complication as any deviation from the normal postoperative course. The Clavien-Dindo classification has gained popularity in many fields of surgery and its use is highly recommended for reporting complications after urologic surgical procedures.[4]

Minor complication: A complication that is inferior in importance, size or degree or is comparatively an unimportant, trivial consequence.

Major complication: A complication that threatens life, damages or endangers an organ partially or completely and deserves remedy.

The Ideal Time for Male Circumcision

The timing of MC is debatable, and it is usually decided based on religious or traditional factors or on non-evidence-based studies, as many social, medical and practical considerations point to the neonatal period as the ideal time for MC, claiming that the neonate is less mobile and amenable to any intervention with low surgical complications and that the health benefits conferred begin immediately. There are different studies recommending different ages for MC, depending on a small number of studied cases and mostly without control samples.

Although a lot of evidence exist about the benefits of MC, it is essential to ask whether these dictate infant MC rather than MC later in life when a boy can make up his own mind. Some of the advantages of MC in infancy were featured in a report from an expert consultation conducted by the US Centers for Disease Control and Prevention (CDC) in 2007.[4]

Actually, the idea of practising circumcision in neonatal period generally and in the first week specifically is a Jewish one. Ancient Egyptians were doing circumcision at adolescence; for Muslims, there is no specific time for performing circumcision, but it just should be done before puberty; and till now, many African tribes practise MC just before marriage, so as to educate the youth for adulthood, although modernity is going against the timing and knowledge inculcated (Figs. 1.3–1.5).

In Turkey the more educated the parents are, the greater the rate of hospital circumcision and older age circumcision, the rate at 2–6 years was 45.9%.[5]

The CDC pointed to an observational study that found the first week post partum to be the best time for MC because pain using local anaesthesia is negligible at this age.[6]

The WHO guidelines mentioned that circumcision is safer for newborns and infants than for older children, noting that the complication rate rises from 0.5% in newborns to 9% in children aged 1–9 years, according to the CDC. Minor bleeding and post MC pain are the most common problems, but I think this is not true, as complications in neonates are usually not encountered or documented in many countries. This is because most circumcisions are done in outpatient clinics or premises, and as most cases are not followed up, many late complications are not accounted. But circumcision in adults is usually done in hospitals and under general anaesthesia, so any minor complications are usually reported and published.

In some communities, groups of boys are circumcised at the same time by a traditional circumciser who uses a traditional technique without anaesthesia. This group activity coincides with the 'rites of passage' from adolescence to adulthood and often takes place in circumcision 'camps' or ceremonies. Circumcision practice is prevalent among the Yao ethnic group in Malawi, where the ceremony takes place between July and September each year and is performed on boys aged 8–13 years. There are many reports of high complication rates following traditional circumcision ceremonies and the circumcisions performed by traditional providers. Safety can be improved by introducing medical circumcision into traditional ceremonies or by performing circumcision under local anaesthesia in a clinic separate from, but linked to, the traditional ceremony. Also, the glamour associated with traditional circumcision and the esteem accorded by traditional circumcisers are matters that need attention before a health clinic is used for MC.

CERTAIN POINTS SHOULD BE CONSIDERED ABOUT THE APPROPRIATE TIME OF PERFORMING MALE CIRCUMCISION
Neonatal Circumcision and Napkin Dermatitis

Many complications may arise after circumcising a neonate, who is still in napkins, especially in developing countries where proper napkin care is not applicable and the frequency of napkin changes is dominated by the economic and social standards (Fig. 1.6).

Different types of napkin dermatitis and rashes, contact, fungal or bacterial dermatitis, are known to complicate MC in a countless number of neonates in developing countries, but this is neither documented nor reported because there is no long-term follow-up for neonates after MC and most of the mothers in developing countries will not seek any medical advice after commencing MC, assuming that the baby has been purified after getting rid of the dirty sinful prepuce, as they usually consider the act of circumcision as a measure of moral hygiene (Fig. 1.7).

Napkin dermatitis may result in different forms of balanitis and balanoposthitis, especially if the circumcision is incomplete, as well as in meatitis, meatal ulcers and meatal stenosis, which, if not detected early and treated properly, may subsequently lead to an ascending UTI (Fig. 1.8).

There is a confusion, even in developed countries, regarding the proper care and hygienic practices for both the circumcised and the uncircumcised penis. The lack of guidance from healthcare providers may be due to a lack of consensus about the proper care of the prepuce, when to begin and how often to retract the foreskin or its remnants or when phimosis requires treatment.[7]

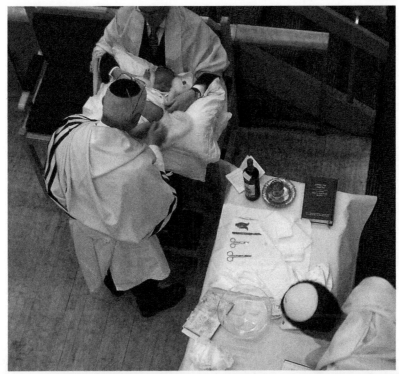

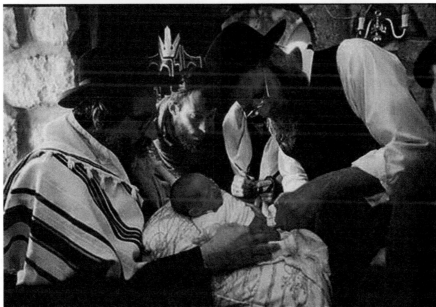

FIG. 1.3 Preparing for a Jewish ritual circumcision for a neonate at the eighth day.

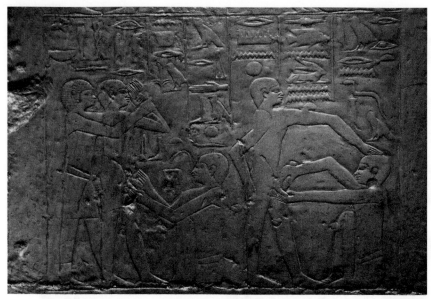

FIG. 1.4 Ancient Egyptian male circumcision at adolescence. This bas-relief from the Egyptian necropolis at Saqqara (c. 2400 BCE) is the world's most ancient depiction of a surgical operation. (Wellcome Institute Library: https://wellcomelibrary.org/.)

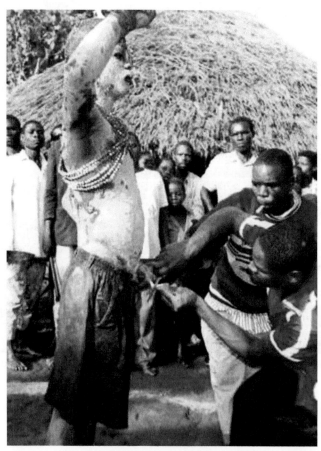

FIG. 1.5 Adolescent circumcision in Africa.

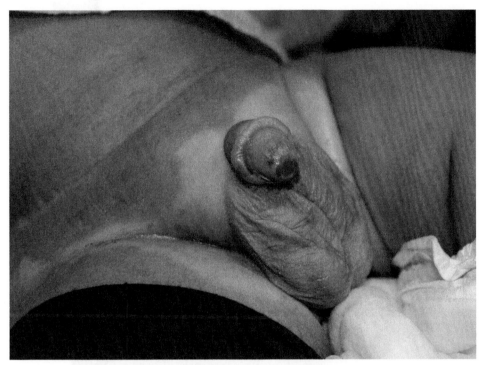

FIG. 1.6 Severe napkin dermatitis after neonatal circumcision.

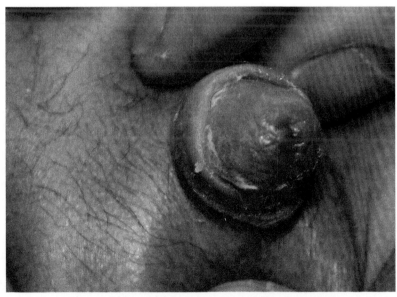

FIG. 1.7 A circumcised neonate with balanitis and meatitis.

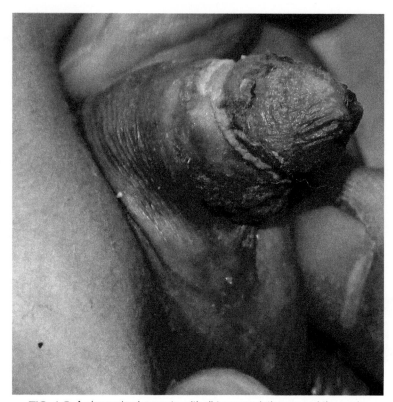

FIG. 1.8 A circumcised neonate with dirt accumulation around the penis.

Neonatal Circumcision and Coagulation Status

There is a belief among gynaecologists and general practitioners that MC should be performed in the first week of life to get the maximum benefit of the maternally transmitted coagulation factors, and not to postpone it to avoid the transient deficiency of these factors, which occurs after the first week of life, but this was proved to be a false belief, as normal babies could be circumcised or even operated at any time.

Neonatal Circumcision and Prematurity

In many countries, and as a regard of false belief of the mandate to circumcise the baby at the eighth day or at least during the neonatal period, we are seeing many preterm babies or those of low birth weight circumcised at this critical situation, and this usually results in a higher rate of complications, mainly the infectious ones.

Sometimes MC is performed to premature babies even in the developed countries, especially in the United States, as the families insist to have the baby circumcised before discharge from the hospital. Also,

some enthusiastic physicians may recommend MC for preterm babies, assuming the protective role of MC against UTI, which had a high incidence of complications in preterm infants. Circumcision guidelines recommend not to circumcise premature infants because of their fragile health status.[8]

Neonatal Circumcision and Anaesthesia

Most centers and publications recommending neonatal circumcision claim, on a nonscientific basis and without any sort of controlled or comparative study, that a neonate's perception of pain is less than that of an older baby. Neonates should be circumcised with at least a local anaesthetic and should receive proper post-procedure analgesics.

Neonatal Circumcision and the Parents' Rights to Consent for the Procedure

Opponents to circumcision point out that hospital personnel request parents to make a decision about circumcision, which may imply their belief that the procedure is beneficial. Doctors contend they circumcise male babies because parents request it, whereas parents choose it because doctors advice it. Overall, communication between physicians and parents about circumcision is often insufficient for informed consent, largely because of the emotional discomfort with the subject. The discussion may instead include incorrect tacit assumptions by the doctor and parents about what the other really wants or means. Although doctors do not require that parents choose circumcision, and parents believe they are freely making their own choice, doctors do exercise control over the parents' decisions by controlling information and sometimes making a recommendation. So many modest opponents of MC recommend postponing the procedure until adolescence and the pros and cons of MC to be explained to the young man and to let him to decide about cutting or leaving his foreskin.[9]

REFERENCES

1. Wiswell TE. Circumcision — an update. *Curr Probl Pediatr.* 1992;10:424—431.
2. Earp BD, Allareddy V, Allareddy V, Rotta AT. Factors associated with early deaths following neonatal male circumcision in the United States. *Clinical Pediatrics.* 2001—2010;57(13):1532—1540. https://doi.org/10.1177/0009922818790060.
3. Mitropoulos D, Artibani W, Graefen M, Remzi M, Rouprêt M, Truss M. Reporting and grading of complications after urologic surgical procedures: an ad hoc EAU guidelines panel assessment and recommendations. European Association of Urology Guidelines Panel. *Eur Urol.* 2012;61(2):341—349 [PubMed].
4. Smith DK, Taylor A, Kilmarx PH, et al. Male circumcision in the United States for the prevention of HIV infection and other adverse health outcomes: Report from a CDC consultation. *Publ Health Rep.* 2010;125(Suppl 1):72—82.
5. Sahin F, Beyazova U, Akturk A. Attitudes and practices regarding circumcision in Turkey. *Child Care Health Dev.* 2003;29:275—280. https://doi.org/10.1046/j.1365-2214.2003.00342.x.
6. Banieghbal B. Optimal time for neonatal circumcision: an observation-based study. *J Pediatr Urol.* 2009;5:359—362. https://doi.org/10.1016/j.jpurol.2009.01.002. PMID: 19223238.
7. Li B, Shannon R, Malhotra NR, Rosoklija I, Liu DB. Advising on the care of the uncircumcised penis: A survey of pediatric urologists in the United States. *J Pediatr Urol.* 2018. https://doi.org/10.1016/j.jpurol.2018.05.024 (in press).
8. Wiswell TE, Tencer HL, Welch CA, Chamberlain JL. Circumcision in children beyond the neonatal period. *Pediatrics.* 1993;92:791—793.
9. Burgu B, Aydogdu O, Tangal S, Soygur T. Circumcision: pros and cons. *Indian J Urol.* 2010;26(1):12—15. https://doi.org/10.4103/0970-1591.60437.

CHAPTER 2

Male Circumcision: Historical and Religious Background

ATIENO KILI K'ODHIAMBO, PhD

ABSTRACT

The chapter analyses the historical and religious perspectives of non-therapeutic male circumcision as a phenomenon that may be prone to abuse and contends that the cultures and debatable scientific evidence which support the practice are not sustainable in the light of knowledge explosion occasioned by the internet and human rights movements. On the other hand, therapeutic male circumcision is scientifically sound and acceptable since it is based on true knowledge and understanding.

KEYWORDS

Analysis; History; Human rights movements; Non-therapeutic; Religion; Therapeutic.

INTRODUCTION

In any discipline, the invaluable role of history cannot be underestimated. History provides the vantage point from which different human practices emerge, specifically explaining how humans have moved through time. Apart from explaining the past, history highlights the present situation and provides a framework to envisage the future. It is therefore imperative that historical background to any human activity deserves attention so as to provide a discourse of holistic and educative nature.

This chapter gives a short historical and religious background of male circumcision by tracing the origin of the practice, explaining the present situation and providing some hypothesis for the future. It does not focus on female circumcision, which is sometimes termed female genital mutilation (FGM) or clitoridectomy, a procedure involving the removal of the clitoris or a part of it. Several organizations in the world talk against FGM. Feminist movements condemn FGM, and some countries, such as Kenya, have enacted laws banning the practice.

Human history and religion sometimes go hand in hand and in discussing an issue like male circumcision, it is difficult to leave either out. History looks at human activities in social, political and economic spheres. Religion provides a component of social history where circumcision falls. Economic history incorporates medical issues. The ultimate reality is that all disciplines are interrelated and male circumcision is definitely connected to all human activities.

HISTORICAL AND RELIGIOUS BACKGROUND TO MALE CIRCUMCISION

Male circumcision means generally the removal of the foreskin or the prepuce of the penis.[1] When and why this practice started is debatable. Archaeological evidence points out that human beings emerged on the Earth's surface some 1.5 million years ago and Africa is regarded as the cradle of humankind.[2] Geologically, Africa is the oldest continent. Circumcision started before written history, and probably all communities of the world initially practised circumcision.[3] The Luo of Kenya probably abandoned circumcision in the course of their migration when they learnt that the foreskin provided an important pouch for hiding seeds of valuable crops such as sesame, sorghum and finger millet.[4] So during tribal conflicts, the Luo could easily move on and escape with the seeds, without the seeds being confiscated by their enemies, thus perpetuating their agricultural activities and supply of food on any new land they landed. When tracing the origin of male circumcision, the birth place of humankind and the oldest world continent are important starting points. Nevertheless, human civilizations in which male circumcision is slotted are recent phenomena, but we can say with certainty that Africa is the cradle of circumcision.

Circumcision is a widespread practice in the world.[3] In most traditional circumstances, it is done without recourse to scientific rationale. Apart from Africa, it is

Complications in Male Circumcision. https://doi.org/10.1016/B978-0-323-68127-8.00002-8

practised by the people of the Middle East, Australia (Aborigines), Pacific Islanders and Native Americans (South and North). For people who practice it, it definitely runs in their psyche and eliminating it may, somehow, require vigorous reeducation that alters the personality of an individual. Changes occasioned by modernity may play a big role in altering the whole situation in the future.

Historians attribute the origin of male circumcision to Egypt (Nile Valley), whose civilization flourished between 4000 and 1000 BCE.[5] Circumcision is estimated to have started there about 4000 years ago. As circumcision predates written history, no one knows exactly when it started. Contrastingly, Mesopotamia (the land of Euphrates and Tigris Rivers, which are the present-day Iraq) whose civilization started a bit earlier and flourished between 5000 and 3500 BCE does not have evidence of circumcision. Mesopotamia is the first cradle of world civilization, followed by Egypt, India (Indus Valley) and China (Hwang Ho Valley).

From its origin in Egypt about 4000 years ago, circumcision spread to many African tribes and to the adherents of religions such as Taoism, Hinduism, Judaism and Islam. Abraham who lived between 20th and 19th century BCE is one of the fathers of Judaism, and historians suggest that Abraham and later his Jews tribe lived in Egypt and probably learnt circumcision from there.[6] Judaism, Islam and Christianity are regarded as Abrahamic religions. The Jews lived in Egypt as slaves and they were rescued by Moses who lived around 1200 BCE. Two questions are pertinent to this discussion: Why did the Egyptians circumcise their males? Did God command Abraham to institute circumcision to himself and also to his male offspring or was circumcision learnt from the Egyptians?

The first question hinges heavily on history and the second question on religion. The questions can be attempted by historians, anthropologists and philosophers, although the answers may not be exhaustive. During the Egyptian civilization, in which pharaohs ruled, the government was both secular and theocratic. Priests were the custodians of both secular and religious knowledge and they played a significant role in offering sacrifices to the Egyptian gods.[5,7] Priests were expected to be pure morally and in physical appearance. The presence of the foreskin was regarded as a sign of female sexual organ and impurity and hence it was to be removed. As purity was a status of higher rank and a coveted attribute, the practice of circumcision, which originally was prescribed for the priests, ultimately became adapted by all men.

For the Jews, it is difficult to dispute the idea that male circumcision was ordained by God as attested by the Bible (Genesis 17:10−14), yet in the New Testament as demonstrated by the Council of Jerusalem in the Acts of the Apostles 15, circumcision is not mandatory. It is equally difficult to deny the fact that Jews might have borrowed the practice of male circumcision from their Egyptian masters. The difficulties inherent in the discussion are good because they stimulate further research. Some authorities suggest man's sexual desire as a reason that might have prompted God to command Abraham and his male descendants to be circumcised.[8] Sexual desire deprives man the ability to focus on a task and by removing the foreskin the sensitivity of the penis for sexual intercourse is diminished. This is supported by William Harvey (1578−1657), the Englishman who discovered the circulation of blood in the human body; Gabriello Fallopio (1523−1562), who discovered the fallopian tube in women; and two Church Fathers, St. Augustine of Hippo (354−430) and St. Thomas Aquinas (1225−1274). Christian civilization was enhanced by focusing less on human desires of the flesh, and up to now, human progress can be accounted for in terms of abstinence.

When the Greek and Roman civilizations flourished (700 BCE to CE 1453), they did not allow circumcision because it affects the beauty of human body.[3,5] People who were colonized were not allowed to circumcise their male children and a parent who went against this law was put to death. The Greek and Roman civilizations bequeathed to the world the ordered knowledge we have. When Romans conquered Greece in 146 BCE, it perpetuated and modified Greek civilization until its fall in CE 476. After the fall of Rome, the Greco-Roman civilization survived in the Eastern Roman Empire headquartered at Byzantium (Constantinople) until 1453 when it fell to the Ottoman Turks.

The cherished civilization handed down to humanity from Greeks and Romans did not recommend male circumcision. Christianity, which became the guiding light, hand in hand with the Greco-Roman civilization regarded male circumcision as optional.

MALE CIRCUMCISION IN THE CONTEMPORARY WORLD

In the contemporary world, about 25% of the male population practise circumcision and there are those who support the practice and those who do not.[9] The reasons given for either side are, somehow, difficult to harmonize and come up with a consensus. Some males undergo circumcision because the practice is a part of their culture; some are circumcised for therapeutic reasons, whereas others find the practice imposed on them because of some disputable research findings such as prevention of diseases, which include sexually transmissible infections and human immunodeficiency virus/acquired immune deficiency syndrome (HIV/AIDS). It is the view of many people that people should not be driven to carry out mass circumcision because of the money provided by some donors or any other benefit but that the driving force should be authentic scientific evidence. It is not surprising that the influence of a dominant culture is the cause of male circumcision in some communities. Practices of a dominant culture can be imitated by other cultures so people conform to what their neighbours do.

Cultural practices of circumcision incorporate important values that are passed on from generation to generation. The Bantu race, which occupies the greater part of Africa, does practise male circumcision. Among the Bantu, male circumcision is an enjoyable activity that is accompanied by transmission of cultural values and education of the youth, which is tinged with a lot of religious undertones. Such education makes a community cohesive and united in approaching issues of their concern. Traditional circumcisers are highly regarded in African communities that practice male circumcision. Circumcisers are recognized experts and they are well paid for their work. These experts sometimes brag of the greater knowledge they have, which they say far much surpasses the knowledge possessed by those with university degrees.

Religious circumcision is still unaffected in some faiths.[10,11] For example, in Judaism, circumcision is performed by an organized group known as the *mohel*. Circumcision is accompanied by festivities. People may object circumcision, but the activities that go with it might be very attractive to people. Throughout human history, any event that is celebrated has an indelible mark on the minds of people and they can remember it well from generation to generation. This might probably account for one of the reasons why circumcision might be difficult to erase as a social phenomenon. Although Qur'an is silent on circumcision, some Muslims circumcise their male children usually on the seventh day after birth and others extend the practice to females. In Madagascar, male circumcision is mandatory and it is supported by women, who maintain that having sex with a circumcised man is more enjoyable because it lasts much longer. Muslims advocate for circumcision following into the footsteps of the prophet Muhammad who was himself circumcised.

Politics, as a part of history, influences circumcision. The communities that practice circumcision consider themselves politically and socially above the noncircumcising communities. In African communities where the majority is Bantu who practice circumcision, it is not uncommon to hear derogatory nicknames given to people who do not practice circumcision. Some politicians might go to the extent of denouncing the leadership of an uncircumcised person as inconsequential. With more liberalism and democratic institutions coming up in the world, egoistic tendencies of any race or tribe might be misplaced.

One may have his foreskin therapeutically removed. This is undisputable because the decision is supported by the medical doctor's expertise. Different countries have different laws. For example, in South Africa, circumcision for therapeutic reasons is acceptable for all males regardless of their ages and for nontherapeutic reasons, it is only adults who can undergo it so long as they make independent decisions to do so. South Africa permits elective circumcision for adults only.

Circumcision of infant boys is criticized by psychologists who maintain that it has long-lasting effects on human behavior.[12] As explained by psychoanalysts, the Freudian stages of psychosexual development are affected by circumcision trauma, which has a long-lasting effect on the personality of the victim. Doctors who oppose male circumcision cite trauma as one of the reasons why male circumcision should be abolished. The trauma inflicted on the infants through circumcision, as affirmed by psychologists, disrupts the child-mother bond. Some people take cues from the Bible to advocate for infant circumcision. Here, psychology and religion do not agree, but it is more appropriate to accept an idea that is evidenced by science.

With the advent of HIV/AIDS, male circumcision has been recommended as a method of reducing female to male transmission of HIV/AIDS. The truthfulness of this assertion is debatable, especially in Africa where various organizations promote male circumcision. History repudiates unbiased researches and time will definitely tell where the truth lies. Whether some scientific facts pertaining to performing circumcision to stem the spread of HIV/AIDS can be provided through unbiased researches depends on time.

The idea that circumcision can reduce the incidence of HIV/AIDS infection emerged in 1986 in a letter to the New York Journal of Medicine by Valiere Alcena.[13,14] The idea was picked up by medical researchers, and between 2005 and 2007, three researches were carried out in three places in Africa, i.e., Kenya (Kisumu), South Africa (Orange Farm) and Uganda (Rakai), to ascertain the relationship between HIV/AIDS and foreskin. The researches were led by Robert C. Bailey, Bertran Auvert and Ronald H. Grey, respectively. The findings authenticated male circumcision as a procedure for preventing HIV/AIDS transmission. The findings are disputed and they have raised more questions than answers. For example, why downplay the natural functions of the foreskin? Why do doctors tamper with the undiseased human body, which should be within the jurisdiction of human rights? Can circumcision be universally applicable to all males? What is the difference between FGM and male genital mutilation?

One of the questions relates to the trade in human organ that is prohibited under many laws, although illegal trafficking thrives.[15] In Iran, the law permits, with restrictions, the selling of body parts, whereas in Australia and Singapore, payment and compensation for the living donor are allowed. The sale of the foreskin to transnational corporations, such as Advanced Tissue Sciences of San Diego, Organogenesis and BioSurface Technology, was started in the 1980s and it is still going on.[15] One foreskin can fetch about US $3000, but if it is from an infant, it can go up to over US $10,000. The foreskin is used in cosmetic industry in making skin creams that make old people look younger. It is also used in skin grafts for burns, especially the infant foreskin, which is flexible and can be used for years without replacement and it is unlikely to be rejected. Specific questions arise: What if you are duped into male circumcision but your foreskins form a billion dollar industry for some people? Can laws allow males to undergo circumcision so that they sell their foreskins?

THE FUTURE OF MALE CIRCUMCISION

As discussed in the Introduction, history is also concerned with the future. The events that took place in the past, including those that take place in the present, have future bearings. It is the role of history to provide some predictions.

As a result of human rights movements and knowledge explosion due to Internet accessibility, it will be extremely difficult to sustain a practice like male circumcision. Male circumcision is tantamount to adulteration of the natural beauty of the human body. Different professions such as anthropology, philosophy, political science and sociology will seek to be incorporated in making a decision on male circumcision as a human rights issue, and medical personnel will be restricted to dealing with diagnosed diseases. When the Greek and Roman civilizations flourished between 700 BCE and CE 1453, male circumcision was not allowed

even to the conquered people because it interferes with human beauty and this has some relevance for the future at the moment. In 1971, the American Academy of Paediatrics stated that there is no valid reason for circumcision and this has had an impact and will continue to have greater impact for a considerable number of years to come.

Some circumcised people have sued their parents who made them get circumcised. They want to be compensated for the loss. People who promote male circumcision may face numerous litigations. For example, in 2012, a German court outlawed nontherapeutic infant circumcision.[16] A group of doctors known as "Doctors Opposing Male Circumcision" regularly meet to highlight the short- and long-term effects of the practice. To convince 75% of the world population to adapt male circumcision is a task fraught with obstacles and will not be won.

With the knowledge explosion as a result of the Internet, it may be difficult for a community to adhere to any cultural practice. Communities that gain some educational value from male circumcision may not find it possible to contain the practice because human beings are rapidly moving to a global village where any information spreads fast to everyone. People are rapidly becoming cosmopolitan and cultural practices are changing. Movement of people from one place to another disrupts all social institutions, including circumcision. The people who were brought up in urban centers may have loose connection with traditional practices such as circumcision.

CONCLUSION

Male circumcision is supported by both traditional and conventional approaches. Traditional approaches are culturally rooted, whereas conventional approaches lean heavily on medicine. The approaches face challenges that are controversial and may not result in universal acceptability of the practice. Therapeutic male circumcision might have a brighter future than other types of circumcision.

PROFESSIONAL PROFILE

Dr. Atieno Kili K'Odhiambo taught History and Religion for several years in secondary schools and colleges of teacher education. He is currently a senior lecturer in philosophy of education at the Department of Educational Foundations, University of Nairobi, Kenya. He is a consultant in Special Needs Education. He has published in the areas of education and circumcision. He is a member of the Philosophy of Education Society of

Great Britain (PESGB) and the International Network of Philosophers of Education (INPE).

REFERENCES

1. Tierney J. Circumcision. In: *Catholic Encyclopedia.* Available from: http://www.newadvent.org/cathen/03777a.htm.
2. Wayman E. *How Africa Became the Cradle of Humankind*; 2011. Retrieved from: https://www.smithsonian.com.
3. Cox G, Morris B. *Why Circumcision: From Prehistory to the Twenty-First Century.* 2012 https://doi.org/10.1007/978-1-4471-2858-8_21.
4. K'Odhiambo AK. *The Truth About Male Circumcision: Its Disadvantages Exposed*; 2017. Retrieved from: http:www.ijessnet.com/wp-content/uploads/2017/05/Book.pdf.
5. Nielson PI. *The Origins of Circumcision*; April 23, 2010. Retrieved from: http://suite101.com/a/origins-and-purposes-of-male circumcision.
6. McClellan M. *Abraham and the Chronology of Ancient Mesopotamia*; September 30, 2012. Retrieved from: www.answersingenesis.org.
7. Dogon Creation Myth. (n.d.). Retrieved from: www.bibliotecapleyades.net/mitos_creacion/esp_mitoscreacion_1.htm.
8. Clark A. *Desire: A History of European Sexuality.* New York: Routledge; 2008.
9. Ball P. *Losses From Circumcision*; 2003. Retrieved from: http://www.norm.uk.org/circumcision-lost.html.
10. Collier R. Vital or vestigial? The foreskin has its fans and foes. *Can Med Assoc J.* 2011;183(17):1963–1964. https://doi.org/10.1503/cmaj.109-4014.
11. Ellwood RS, Alles GD. *The Encyclopedia of World Religions.* New York: Facts on File; 2007.
12. Cansever G. Psychological effects of circumcision. *Br J Med Psychol.* 1995;38:321–331.
13. *Doctors Opposing Circumcision*; 2009. Retrieved from: www.doctorsopposingcircumcision.org.
14. Fleiss PM. *Where Is My Foreskin? the Case against Circumcision. Mothering (The Magazine of Natural Family Living)*; Winter 1997. Retrieved from: www.foreskin.org.
15. Yosomono E. *The Bizarrely Profitable Business of Baby Foreskins*; 2013. Retrieved from: http://www.knowledgenuts.com.
16. Levey GB. Thinking about infant male circumcision after the Cologne court decision. *Global Discourse.* 2013;3(2):326–331. Retrieved from: https://doi.org/10.1080/23269995.2013.804765.

CHAPTER 3

Benefits of Male Circumcision (Circumcision Apparition)

MOHAMED A BAKY FAHMY, MD, FRCS

ABSTRACT

It is easy to recognize the bias and its degree in most of the published papers on either the benefits or risks of male circumcision. The decision of an adult or a young man to be circumcised, and the decision of a parent to have his or her son circumcised, should be based on cultures, religion, personal preference and evidence-based information provided by a healthcare worker.

KEYWORDS

Balanitis; Baptism; HIV prevention; Tribal mark.

Along the history of humankind, male circumcision (MC) has been appreciated as
- A tribal mark;
- A mark of nobility and superiority;
- Having a religious significance;
- Giving cleanliness, freedom from disease, offspring and purity of heart;
- A sign of the covenant;
- An initiation into manhood;
- A necessary means of salvation;
- A figure of baptism;
- An indication to the spiritual effect of the sacrament;
- A means of restraining concupiscence.

A review from Canada summarized the reasons for neonatal/childhood circumcision as follows[1]:
- Religious.
- Ethnocultural.
- Social/personal and family values.
- Medical: Cases of phimosis not responding to topical steroids, balanitis xerotica obliterans, paraphimosis, recurrent urinary tract infections (UTIs) and during surgery for some genitourinary anomalies.
- Others: Parents want to prevent diseases at adulthood.

BIASES IN STUDIES

In the past few decades, facing increased scrutiny from legal theorists and medical ethicists, as well as criticism from human rights advocates, supporters of circumcision have sought to revive the 'medical benefits' narrative, casting the procedure as a secularly defensible measure of individual and public health, as opposed to solely a religious practice.[2]

The breakthrough came from the evidence of three randomized controlled trials (RCTs) carried out in the early 2000s in sub-Saharan Africa.[3–5]

These RCTs provided evidence that voluntary circumcision of adult men may reduce the risk of female-to-male human immunodeficiency virus (HIV) transmission in areas with high rates of such heterosexual transmission and a low baseline prevalence of circumcision.

In light of such thinking, mass circumcision as a strategy for HIV/AIDS control is now in full swing throughout the African continent, with the generous backing of American funders.

It is easy to recognize the bias and its degree in most of the published papers on either the benefits or risks of MC.

The Manual for Male Circumcision under Local Anesthesia, Version 3.1 December 2009, WHO and UNAIDS mentions clearly

'The decision of an adult or young man to be circumcised, and the decision of a parent to have his or her son circumcised, should be based on culture, religion, personal preference, and evidence-based information provided by a health care worker.'

Many publications showed that early infant MC confers immediate and lifelong benefits by protecting against UTIs having potential adverse long-term renal effects, phimosis that causes difficult and painful erections and 'ballooning' during urination, inflammatory skin conditions, inferior penile hygiene, candidiasis, various sexually transmissible infections in both sexes, genital ulcers and penile, prostate and cervical cancers.

Complications in Male Circumcision. https://doi.org/10.1016/B978-0-323-68127-8.00003-X

Risk-benefit analysis showed that benefits exceeded procedural risks, which are predominantly minor, by up to 200 to 1. It is estimated that more than one in two uncircumcised males will experience an adverse foreskin-related medical condition over his lifetime. Wide-ranging evidence from surveys, physiologic measurements and the anatomic location of penile sensory receptors responsible for sexual sensation strongly and consistently suggested that MC has no detrimental effect on sexual function, sensitivity or pleasure. However, studies from the United States showed that early infant MC is cost saving.

The evidence supporting early infant MC has further strengthened since the positive reviews of the American Academy of Pediatrics (AAP) and the Centers for Disease Control and Prevention (CDC).[6–8]

The AAP began an extensive review of the evidence accumulated until 2010. This led to the formulation and release of a new affirmative early infant MC policy statement in 2012, which concluded the following based on the evidence[7]:

1. The benefits of early infant MC exceed risks.
2. Parents should be given factually correct, nonbiased information on MC before conception or early in a pregnancy.
3. Access to MC should be provided routinely for those families who choose it.
4. Education and training should be provided to practitioners to enhance their competency.
5. The procedure should be performed by trained competent practitioners using sterile techniques and effective pain management.
6. The preventive and public health benefits warrant third-party reimbursement.

The American College of Obstetricians and Gynaecologists endorsed these recommendations, and the American Urological Association's website has a brief statement that presents benefits and risks of infant MC.[8]

Bennett et al.[9] demonstrated with highly statistical significance that a relationship exists between epididymitis and the presence of a foreskin, as they found that an intact foreskin is an important etiologic factor in boys with epididymitis. Acute epididymitis in prepubertal male individuals is uncommon but it represents an important consideration in the differential diagnosis of acute scrotal swelling.

Bossio[10] studied 62 men between the ages of 18 and 37 years, among whom 30 were circumcised and 32 were not. Four penile sites were tested using touch, pain, warmth detection and heat pain. The results indicated that neonatal circumcision is not associated with changes in penile sensitivity and provided evidence to suggest the foreskin is not the most sensitive part of the penis.

According to a study by the University of Sydney, Penile cancer, HIV, human papilloma virus (HPV) infection, syphilis and kidney inflammation are among a number of medical conditions whose risk can be lowered by the practice of infant MC.

The review of current international evidence for the benefits and risks of infant MC has been published in the Open Journal of Preventive Medicine: "This is the world's first evidence-based policy on infant circumcision and its authors include five Fellows of the Royal Australasian College of Physicians" The lead author, Professor Brian Morris, from Sydney Medical School said, "The evidence in favor of infant circumcision is now so strong that advocating this simple, inexpensive procedure for baby boys is about as effective and safe as childhood vaccination".

The study points out that many common childhood conditions, including kidney damage, will become rare if baby boys are circumcised in the first weeks of life. Circumcision was found to protect men, and their sexual partners, from several common sexually transmitted infections (STIs), as well as from cancers of the penis and cervix. "The scientific evidence shows no adverse effects on sexual function, sensitivity, satisfaction or sensation — if anything the opposite," said Professor Morris.

The policy suggests that for maximum benefits, safety, convenience and cost savings, circumcision should be performed in infancy and with local anaesthesia. It claims that the risk-benefit analysis shows benefits outweigh minor risks by a factor of over 100 to 1.

It is now up to state governments to ensure that bans on elective infant MC in public hospitals are lifted without delay, and it is essential that the federal government revises the Medicare rebate so that this procedure is affordable for low-income families.

It is reasonable for parents to weigh the benefits and risks of circumcision and to make the decision whether or not to circumcise their sons. The policy recommended that 'when parents request a circumcision for their child, the medical attendant is obliged to provide accurate unbiased and up to date information on the risks and benefits of the procedure'. It also stated that 'parental choice should be respected' and that, the operation, 'should be undertaken in a safe, child-friendly environment by an appropriately trained competent practitioner, capable of dealing with the complications, and using appropriate analgesia'.

A brief statement placed on the Internet by the Royal Colleges covering surgeons, nurses, paediatricians and anaesthetists in the United Kingdom in 2000 did not claim to be evidence based and only mentions MC for treatment of phimosis, balanoposthitis and 'some rare conditions'. The policy of the Royal Dutch Medical Association in 2010 states that 'non-therapeutic circumcision of male minors is a violation of children's rights to autonomy and physical integrity'. It refers only to the 'complications' of the procedure and urges 'a strong policy of deterrence'. The recent policy statements by the AAP, CDC, Circumcision Academy of Australia (CAA) and even the Canadian Paediatric Society (CPS) have raised the bar, meaning statements by other bodies should now be expected to similarly consider the evidence rather than rely on opinions.

RECOMMENDATIONS (MALE CIRCUMCISION AND PREVENTION OF URINARY TRACT INFECTION)

1. Neonatal circumcision decreases the risk of UTI.
2. The risk of UTI is low in infant males and decreases further beyond infancy.
3. There is paucity of level 1 evidence to justify recommending universal circumcision to prevent UTIs in normal males.
4. A stronger effect of neonatal circumcision in preventing UTIs in boys with urologic abnormalities has been demonstrated, and therefore it is recommended that a discussion with the parents is advisable for this subgroup of neonates.
   The costs saved will be enormous, as this policy statement shows that half of the uncircumcised males will suffer an adverse medical condition over their lifetime, and many will die as a result of diseases preventable by circumcision.
5. MC significantly reduces the bacterial colonization of the glans penis with regard to both non-uropathogenic and uropathogenic bacteria.[11]

CIRCUMCISION AND BALANITIS

Meta-analysis of balanitis and circumcision status of eight relevant studies found that prevalence of balanitis was 68% lower in circumcised versus uncircumcised males (odds ratio = 0.32; 95% confidence interval [CI], 0.20–0.52), i.e., 3.1 times (95% CI, 1.9–5.0) higher in uncircumcised males.[12]

Circumcision of males, particularly early in life, substantially reduced the risk of penile inflammatory conditions. The clinical and personal burden of penile inflammatory conditions in males can be ameliorated by preventive measures, most notably circumcision.

CIRCUMCISION AND PREVENTION OF HUMAN IMMUNODEFICIENCY VIRUS INFECTION

The Canadian guidelines on the care of the normal foreskin and neonatal circumcision reached to the following conclusions[1]:

1. With respect to HIV infection prevention, MC is one of the several partially effective risk-reduction alternatives for heterosexual men, which should be used in combination with other measures.
2. There is no need or equipoise to conduct a US trial of MC for HIV infection prevention among men who have sex with women.
3. There is not enough evidence to make a recommendation for MC in men who have sex with men (MSM) to prevent HIV infection, and there may be equipoise to conduct an efficacy trial for this population.
4. For newborns, medical benefits outweigh risks, and the benefits and risks should be explained to parents.

MALE CIRCUMCISION AND ULCERATIVE SEXUALLY TRANSMITTED INFECTIONS

Currently, there is no significant evidence to support the protective role of universal neonatal circumcision for males and females in the acquisition of ulcerative STIs (Level 2–4 evidence, Grade C recommendation). There is weak evidence of decreased seroconversion for herpes simplex virus type 2 following MC in adult men in Africa (Level 2a–b).[13]

CIRCUMCISION AND RISK OF PENILE CANCER

This will be discussed in detail in Chapter 4; however, it is difficult to justify universal neonatal circumcision as a preventive strategy for preventing penile cancer.

Recognition and treatment of phimosis during regular health visits is generally recommended to decrease the risk of penile cancer. A genitourinary examination during puberty is recommended to ensure preputial retractability and hygiene, to rule out phimosis and to counsel regarding HPV vaccination, safe sexual practices and the possibility of circumcision as a preventive measure against STIs while specifying the drawbacks and efficacy of other preventive measures.

CIRCUMCISION AND RISK OF PROSTATE CANCER

There is no convincing evidence on the protective effect of MC against prostate cancer. An international study from the University of North Carolina shows that among Kenyan men, circumcision is associated with a lower prevalence of HPV infection. HPV is a sexually transmitted virus that plays an important role in genital cancers in men and women, including cancers of the penis, prostate and cervix.[13]

For many children or even men, accessing circumcision services may be their first contact with health services, so this contact offers an opportunity to address other aspects of men's sexual and reproductive health and to detect other associated or coincident congenital anomalies; several publications have addressed the incidences of different diseases among children attending hospitals for MC, and this trend should be promoted and financially supported to help in the early detection of congenital anomalies in children and other acquired sexual problems in adults.

CIRCUMCISION AND ITS EFFECT ON SEXUAL BEHAVIOUR

The relationship between the practice of circumcision and sexual behaviour of males appears to be more complex than could be explained by a cause and effect relationship. In a study utilizing the Demographic and Health Surveys of 11 priority countries in East Africa, Lau et al.[14] reported that circumcised men were more likely to engage in risky sexual behaviour (adjusted odds ratio [aOR] = 1.65; 95% CI, 1.58–1.73) and had sexual debut before the age of 14 years (aOR = 1.72; 95% CI, 1.47–2.00). Although these differences were not seen in unadjusted regional results, in this study, respondents with higher levels of education and higher socioeconomic status were more likely to be circumcised.[7]

REFERENCES

1. Abara EO. Prepuce health and childhood circumcision: choices in canada. *Can Urol Assoc J.* 2017;11(1–2S). https://doi.org/10.5489/cuaj.4447.
2. Earp, BD, Darby, R. *Circumcision, Autonomy, and Public Health.* Public Health Ethics. http://www.researchgate.net/publication/320853591.
3. Auvert B, Sobngwi-Tambekou J, Cutler E, et al. Effect of male circumcision o the prevalence of high-risk human papillomavirus in young men: results of a randomized controlled trial conducted in Orange Farm, South Africa. *J Infect Dis.* 2009;199(1):14–19.
4. Bailey RC, Nyaboke I, Otieno FO. What device would be best for early infant male circumcision in East and Southern Africa? Provider experiences and opinions with three different devices in Kenya. *PLoS One.* 2017;12:e0171445. https://doi.org/10.1371/journal.pone.0171445.
5. Gray RH, Kigozi G, Serwadda D, et al. Male circumcision for HIV prevention in men in Rakai, Uganda: a randomised trial. *Lancet.* 2007;369(9562):657–666. PMID: 17321311.
6. Morris BJ, Kennedy SE, Wodak AD, et al. Early infant male circumcision: systematic review, risk-benefit analysis, and progress in policy. *World J Clin Pediatr.* 2017;6(1): 89–102. http://www.wjgnet.com/2219-2808/full/v6/i1/89.htm.
7. American Academy of Pediatrics task force on circumcision: male circumcision. *Pediatrics.* 2012;130:e756–e785. PMID: 22926175.
8. American Urological Association. Circumcision. Available from: http://www.auanet.org/about/policy-statements/circumcision.cfm.
9. Bennett RT, Gill B, Kogan S. Epididymitis in children: the circumcision factor? *J Urol.* 1998;160:1842–1844.
10. Bossio JA, et al. Examining penile sensitivity in neonatally circumcised and intact men using quantitative sensory testing. *J Urol.* 2015. https://doi.org/10.1016/j.juro.2015.12.080.
11. Ladenhauf HN, Ardelean MA, Schimke C, Yankovic F, Schimpl G. Reduced bacterial colonisation of the glans penis after male circumcision in children–a prospective study. *J Pediatr Urol.* 2013;9(6 Pt B):1137–1144. https://doi.org/10.1016/j.jpurol.2013.04.011.
12. Morris BJ, Krieger JN. Penile inflammatory skin disorders and the preventive role of circumcision. *Int J Prev Med.* 2017;8:32. PMC Web 31 July 2018.
13. WHO/UNAIDS. *Male Circumcision: Global Trends and Determinants of Prevalence, Safety and Acceptability.* Geneva: World Health Organization; 2008.
14. Lau FK, Jayakumar S, Sgaier SK. Understanding the socioeconomic and sexual behavioural correlates of male circumcision across eleven voluntary medical male circumcision priority countries in Southeastern Africa. *BMC Public Health.* 2015;15:813.

CHAPTER 4

Circumcision and Penile Cancer

ANTHONY EMMANUEL, BSc (Hons), DipRD, MD (Res), MRCS (Eng) •
NICK WATKIN, MA, MChir, FRCS (Urol)

ABSTRACT

Penile cancer is a rare malignancy, with wide variation in its global incidence rates and health burden. Multiple risk factors are linked to this debilitating disease and possible preventative strategies are well documented. Circumcision is one such strategy and has been shown to prevent this rare and potentially debilitating disease from occurring due to the improved penile hygiene, lower HPV and HIV transmission rates and reduction of chronic inflammatory conditions such as phimosis and balanitis. Although, whether circumcision should be advocated in all males to harness its multi-faceted benefits is controversial and currently, with no official recommendation, the decision will ultimately lie with parents and/or the patient.

KEYWORDS

Balanitis; Circumcision; Human papilloma virus; Neonatal circumcision; Penile cancer.

INTRODUCTION

Penile cancer is a rare malignancy with wide variations in its global incidence rates and health burden. Multiple risk factors are linked to this debilitating disease and possible preventative strategies are well documented, of which with incipient controversy and ongoing debate, circumcision has been advocated. This chapter aims to explore the relationship between circumcision and penile cancer.

PENILE CANCER: EPIDEMIOLOGY AND RISK FACTORS

Briefly, penile cancer is a rare disease in the western world, with an overall incidence of <1 per 100,000 men.[1] However, this figure is significantly higher in developing countries such as Brazil and Uganda, with rates up to 3−6.8 per 100,000 men.[2] This malignancy occurs predominantly in elderly men, with an increasing incidence with age and the highest rate being between 50 and 70 years.[3]

Penile tumours, of which 95% are squamous cell carcinoma, originate most commonly from the epithelium of the penile glans, inner prepuce (foreskin) and coronal sulcus and less commonly on the penile shaft[3−5] (Fig. 4.1).

Several risk factors have been identified, which are thought to contribute to the development of penile cancer. One of the most important and extensively studied factor is infection with the human papilloma virus (HPV). Around 33% of all penile cancer cases are associated with HPV infection, similar to vulvar and head and neck cancers.[4−7] Other risk factors include phimosis, chronic inflammation, poor penile hygiene, penile trauma, ultraviolet A photochemotherapy, multiple sexual partners and smoking. There is no evidence that smegma is carcinogenic.[8] However, with poor penile hygiene, its prolonged presence within the prepuce may cause penile irritation and inflammation, which may increase the risk of penile cancer.[7,9,10]

THE RELATIONSHIP BETWEEN CIRCUMCISION AND PENILE CANCER

Circumcision, a long-standing practice that predates human history, is one if not the most common suprocedures performed worldwide. It is usually carried out to treat an underlying physiologic phimosis or a pathologic phimosis caused by traumatic injury or balanitis xerotica obliterans, refractory balanoposthitis, chronic, recurrent urinary tract infections, etc.[10,11] In addition, it may be performed for religious (Jewish and Islamic faith), cultural (for example, Korean, Turkish and African groups) or social reasons.[12]

Circumcision has been widely debated as a preventive measure for urinary tract infections, sexually transmitted infections, human immunodeficiency virus/acquired immunodeficiency syndrome (HIV/AIDS) and penile inflammation. The link between circumcision

Complications in Male Circumcision. https://doi.org/10.1016/B978-0-323-68127-8.00004-1

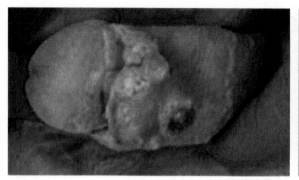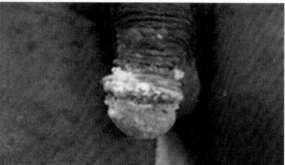

FIG. 4.1 Examples of penile cancer involving the prepuce.

and penile cancer has been well documented, with the lack of circumcision and neonatal circumcision found to be a risk and protective factor, respectively.[13] Owing to these factors, although controversial, some authors have advocated for universal male neonatal circumcision as a means to prevent penile cancer, while no current major medical organization has recommended or reprimanded this practice.

Lack of circumcision is found to be a risk factor of penile cancer because of its association with an increased risk of phimosis and balanitis, which themselves, as shown by meta-analysis, increase the risk of penile cancer by 12- and 4-fold, respectively.[14,15] The prevalence of HPV infection has been shown by several studies to be significantly less in circumcised individuals in comparison to their uncircumcised counterparts. This site-specific effect likely reflects the suitable environment for HPV infection created by the foreskin, as it surrounds the glans penis. Thereby, male circumcision reduces the risk of HPV infection among men and consequently reduces the exposure of women to high-risk HPV infection.[16,17] In addition, multiple studies have shown that circumcised men clear penile oncogenic HPV infection faster than uncircumcised individuals, and this can further explain the lower risk of penile cancer and cervical cancer in female partners.[17]

Despite the obvious benefits of circumcision in reducing the risk of penile inflammatory conditions and HPV and HIV transmission, which can lead to penile cancer, interestingly, the incidence of penile cancer has been found to be similar in the United States and Denmark (∼0.8 per 100,000) that have high and low rates of circumcision, respectively.[18,19] In Denmark, one possible reason attributed to the low incidence of penile cancer despite a low rate of circumcision (<2%

of males) is improved penile hygiene, as the proportion of Danish people dwelling with a bath increased from 35% in 1940 to 90% in 1990.[18]

It has been shown that countries and cultures practising routine neonatal circumcision have a lower incidence of penile cancer. The incidence of penile cancer in the Jewish population, where neonatal circumcision is universally practiced is 0.3/100,000 per year in comparison to India, 3.32/100,000 per year, where neonatal circumcision is not routine.[19]

Neonatal circumcision removes approximately half the tissue that can develop into penile cancer. The protective effect of neonatal circumcision against penile cancer is in its prevention of penile inflammation caused by phimosis, among others. This was exemplified in a study of 100 matched case-control pairs, which compared those who underwent neonatal circumcision with those who were never circumcised and does not have a history of phimosis (odds ratio [OR] 0.41; 95% confidence interval [CI], 0.13−1.1 vs. OR 0.79; 95% CI, 0.29−2.6). This protective effect of circumcision against penile cancer is higher if performed in the neonatal period, and this effect diminishes if performed in later life, but to what extent remains unclear.[20]

There is a clear multi-faceted benefit to circumcision; however, the risks of possible complications, such as bleeding, infection and poor cosmesis, from undergoing this operation need to be considered.[19,21] Other less invasive methods for the prevention of penile cancer do exist and these include following preventative strategies for sexually transmitted infection, such as condom use; promoting good penile hygiene; and HPV vaccination, either directly or from herd immunity from current vaccination programs in developed countries to prevent cervical cancer in women.[21]

SUMMARY

The presence of a foreskin does not increase the risk of penile cancer; however, the presence of phimosis in men with penile carcinoma is high. Circumcision has been shown to prevent this rare and potentially debilitating disease from occurring because of the improved penile hygiene, lower HPV and HIV transmission rates and reduction of chronic inflammatory conditions such as phimosis and balanitis. Whether circumcision should be advocated in all men to harness its multifaceted benefits is controversial, and currently, with no official recommendation, the decision will ultimately lie with parents and/or patients.

REFERENCES

1. Barski D, Georgas E, Gerullis H, et al. Metastatic penile carcinoma — an update on the current diagnosis and treatment options. *Cent European J Urol.* 2014;67(2): 126—132.

2. Christodoulidou M, Sahdev V, Houssein S, et al. Epidemiology of penile cancer. *Curr Probl Cancer.* 2015;39(3): 126—136.

3. Hakenberg OW, Comperat EM, Minhas S, et al. EAU guidelines on penile cancer: 2014 update. *Eur Urol.* 2014;67(1): 142—150.

4. Barnholtz-Sloan JS, Maldonado JL, Pow-sang J, et al. Incidence trends in primary malignant penile cancer. *Urol Oncol.* 2007;25(5):361—367.

5. Alemany L, Cubilla A, Halec G, et al. Role of human papillomavirus in penile carcinomas worldwide. *Eur Urol.* 2016, May;69(5):953—961.

6. Longpre MJ, Lange PH, Kwon JS, et al. Penile carcinoma: lessons learned from vulvar carcinoma. *J Urol.* 2013; 189(1):17—24.

7. Douglawi A, Masterson TA. Updates on the epidemiology and risk factors for penile cancer. *Transl Androl Urol.* 2017; 6(5):785—790.

8. Van Howe RS, Hodges FM. The carcinogenicity of smegma: debunking a myth. *J Eur Acad Dermatol Venereol.* 2006; 20(9):1046—1054.

9. Krustrup D, Jensen HL, van den Brule AJ, et al. Histological characteristics of human papilloma-virus-positive and -negative invasive and in situ squamous cell tumours of the penis. *Int J Exp Pathol.* 2009;90(2):182—189.

10. Morris BJ, Waskett JH, Banerjee J, et al. A 'snip' in time: what is the best age to circumcise? *BMC Pediatr.* 2012;28: 12—20.

11. Malone P, Steinbrecher H. Medical aspects of male circumcision. *BMJ.* 2007;335(7631):1206—1290.

12. Hayashi Y, Kohri L. Circumcision related to urinary tract infection, sexually transmitted infections, human immunodeficiency virus infections, and penile and cervical cancer. *Int J Urol.* 2013;20(8):769—775.

13. Perera CL, Bridgewater FH, Thavaneswaran P, et al. Safety and efficacy of nontherapeutic male circumcision: a systematic review. *Ann Fam Med.* 2010;8(1):64—72.

14. Larke NL, Thomas SL, dos Santos Silva I, et al. Male circumcision and penile cancer: a systematic review and meta-analysis. *Cancer Causes Control.* 2011;22(8):1097—1110.

15. Morris BJ, Gray RH, Castellsague, et al. The strong protective effect of circumcision against cancer of the penis. *Adv Urol.* 2011;2011:812368.

16. Auvert, Sobngwi-Tambekou J, Cutler E, et al. Effect of male circumcision on the prevalence of high-risk human papillomavirus in young men: results of a randomized controlled trial conducted in Orange Farm, South Africa. *J Infect Dis.* 2009;199(1):14—19.

17. Lu B, Wu Y, Nielson CM, et al. Factors associated with acquisition and clearance of human papillomavirus infection in a cohort of US men: a prospective study. *J Infect Dis.* 2009;199(3):362—371.

18. Frisch M, Friis S, Kjaer SK, et al. Falling incidence of penis cancer in an uncircumcised population (Denmark 1943—90). *BMJ.* 1995;311(7018):1471.

19. Ornellas AA, Ornellas P. Should routine neonatal circumcision be a policy to prevent penile cancer? | Opinion: Yes. *Int Braz J Urol.* 2017;43(1):7—9.

20. Tsen HF, Morgenstern H, Mack T, Peters RK. Risk factors for penile cancer: results of a population-based case-control study in Los Angeles County (United States). *Cancer Causes Control.* 2001;12(3):267—277.

21. Tang DH, Spiess PE. Should routine neonatal circumcision be a policy to prevent penile cancer? | Opinion: No. *Int Braz J Urol.* 2017;43(1):10—12.

CHAPTER 5

Methods and Techniques of Circumcision

MOHAMED A BAKY FAHMY, MD, FRCS

ABSTRACT

Along human history, a wide varieties of methods and tools had been used for male circumcision, and till now, a wide variety of instruments and techniques are used in different countries. Many domestic tools are still in use in many developing countries, especially in rural areas, with an expected higher rate of complications.

KEYWORDS

Circumcision staple; Gomco clamp; Guillotine circumcision; Mogen clamp; Plastibell; Sleeve resection; Smart Klamp; Thermal cutting.

Along human history, a wide varieties of methods and tools had been used for male circumcision (MC), and till now, a wide variety of instruments and techniques are used in different countries (Fig. 5.1). Many domestic tools are still in use in many developing countries, especially in rural areas, with an expected higher rate of complications (Fig. 5.2).

In January 2008, the World Health Organization (WHO) published a long-awaited document describing the different methods of circumcision for both men and boys, along with the issues related to performing this procedure. It is called the Manual for Male Circumcision under Local Anaesthesia and includes an excellent, authoritative overview of the subject of instruments and techniques.[1]

The principles of circumcision are aseptic, adequate excision of the outer and inner preputial skin layers, haemostasis, protection of the glans and urethra and cosmesis. The goal of the procedure is to expose the glans sufficient to prevent phimosis or paraphimosis. Circumcision methods can be classified into the following three major types or combinations:

- Dorsal slit
- Shield and clamp
- Surgical excision

Many methods in use today fall in to one of these major classes. Shield and clamp adopts the use of a device to effect circumcision, obviating the use of knife in majority of cases. The device method is the commonly used method of circumcision in recent practice.

Although there are different studies about the various circumcision methods in the literature, researchers are still debating about the most convenient and the safest circumcision method. The choice of circumcision method depends on the physician's level of confidence and training, and other factors such as the cost of the procedure, medical insurance coverage and teaching program in each country dominate the choice of the procedure. The most commonly utilized techniques in the United States in the newborn nursery setting are the Gomco clamp (Fig. 5.3), Mogen clamp (Fig. 5.4) and Plastibell (Fig. 5.5). Although all these devices can be used in the operating room, 'freehand circumcision' using either the sleeve technique or the dorsoventral slit technique is the most commonly used technique by surgeons in the operating room (Fig. 5.6). Each instrument and technique carries its own benefits and complication risks. The elements that are common to the use of each of these devices to accomplish circumcision include the following:

- Estimation of the amount of external skin to be removed.
- Dilation of the preputial orifice so that the glans can be visualized and secured along the procedure.
- Bluntly freeing the inner preputial epithelium from the epithelium of the glans.
- Placing the device (sometimes a dorsal slit is necessary to do so).
- Leaving the device in situ long enough to produce haemostasis.
- Amputation of the foreskin.

Different other clamps (Smart Klamp, Tara KLamp, etc.), with different techniques but haemostasis usually achieved by means of electrical energy (monopolar, bipolar cautery, thermocautery).[2] Complications of

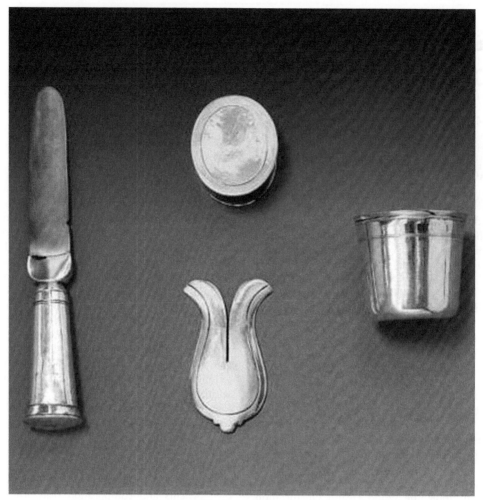

FIG. 5.1 A set of tools used by the mohel for circumcision during 1700s.

thermocautery will be discussed with penile injuries and penile amputation (Chapter 12).

GOMCO CLAMP

This is the oldest and the most refined instrument, it was invented by Dr. Hiram S. Yellen and Aaron A. Goldstein in 1935 (Fig. 5.3).[2] Unlike the Plastibell, this clamp is reusable and precautions are needed to ensure its sterility. The Gomco clamp has different bell sizes and can be used in infants and older children. The foreskin is dorsally crushed with a haemostat, then slit with scissors from the tip to the coronal sulcus done, the foreskin is drawn over the bell-shaped portion of the clamp and inserted through a hole in the base of the clamp and the clamp is tightened, 'crushing the foreskin between the bell and the base plate'. It is supposed that the crushed blood vessels provide haemostasis. The flared bottom of the bell fits tightly against the hole of the base plate, so the foreskin may be cut away with a scalpel from above the base plate.

MOGEN CLAMP

The word 'Mogen' is derived from the Hebrew word for 'shield'. This clamp was introduced by Dr. Harry Bronstein in 1955 (Fig. 5.4). Mogen clamps serve to protect the penis during excising the prepuce. The clamp is used widely in North America and its complications are less frequent than in other methods when used in neonates.

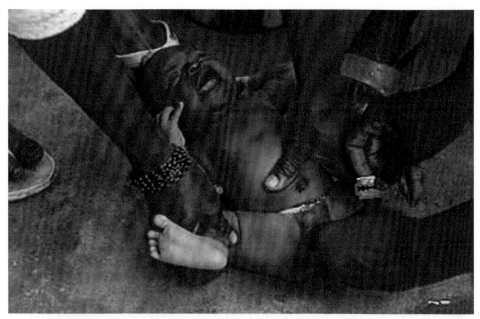

FIG. 5.2 A small baby circumcised using a razor in Africa.

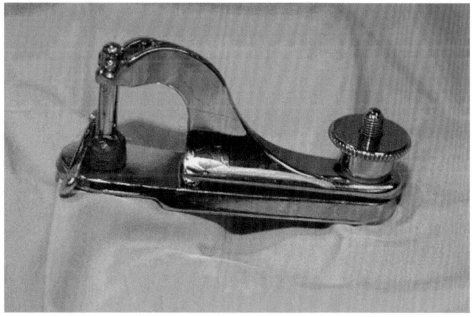

FIG. 5.3 Gomco clamp.

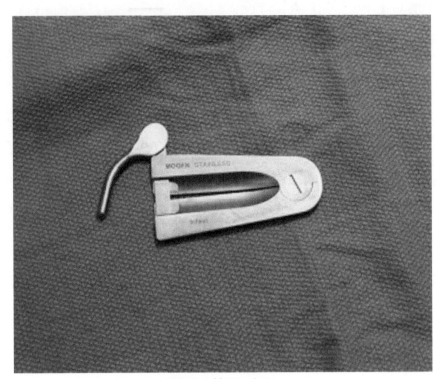

FIG. 5.4 Mogen clamp.

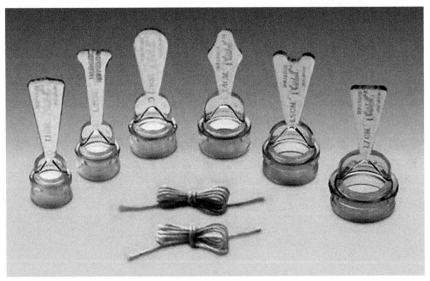

FIG. 5.5 Plastibell clamp.

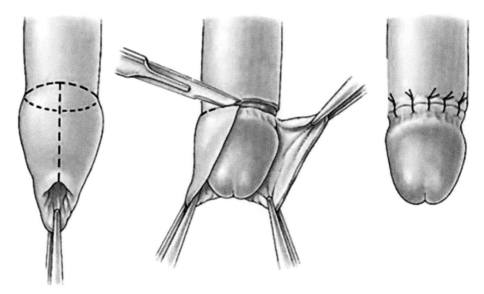

FIG. 5.6 Sleeve technique for male circumcision.

Comparative studies have shown that it is quicker and causes less pain than the Gomco clamp.

The foreskin is pulled dorsally with a straight haemostat and lifted. The Mogen clamp is then slided between the glans and haemostat, following the angle of the corona to 'avoid removing excess skin ventrally and to obtain a superior cosmetic result' than that with Gomco or Plastibell circumcision. The clamp is locked and a scalpel is used to cut the skin from the flat (upper) side of the clamp.[3]

PLASTIBELL

Hollister Inc., USA invented the Plastibell in 1950, but circumcision with Plastibell was first reported in 1953 (Fig. 5.5). Initially, it was called the scalpel-free technique because the preputial skin was not cut, but left to slough off; the Plastibell shedding time ranges from 3 to 8 days.[4]

The Plastibell plastic ring is placed under the foreskin and secured with a circumferential ligature, which prevents bleeding when the distal foreskin is excised. The entire procedure takes 5–10 min. Circumcision with Plastibell is the most popular method among surgeons in the United States and in many Asian countries. It is seldom used in children older than 2 years because of thickening of the preputial skin. Selection of the appropriate size of bell and proper placement over glans is mandatory. The use of local anaesthesia for the procedure is recommended for neonates and older children.

It is safe and has minimal complications with excellent outcome in infants; however, it is associated with significant complications in children older than 1 year.

The complications of Plastibell include the following:
- Proximal migration of the bell.
- Necrotizing fasciitis of the skin of penis.
- Injury to the glans.
- Rupture of the bladder secondary to proximal urinary obstruction.
- Haematoma and affected Plastibell after circumcision.
- Late complications include
  - Wound infection
  - Meatal stenosis
  - phimosis
  - inadequate or overdone circumcision leading to buried penis
  - urethral fistula
  - sepsis.

SMART KLAMP

The removal of the clamp was the most problematic part of the procedure for patients (Fig. 5.7). Although its proponents advise that the clamp can be removed easily with some discomfort, 20% of patients

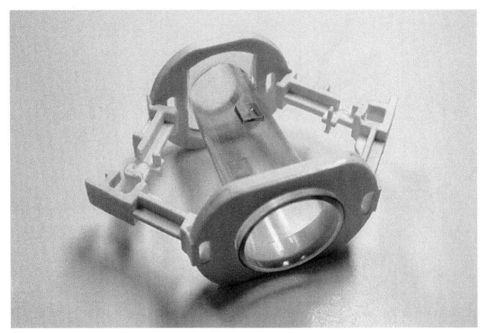

FIG. 5.7 Smart Klamp with different sizes.

complained of complications on removal of the clamp, 14% complained of pain during and after removal and 6% patients had swelling and pus discharge complicating removal of the clamp.[5] For optimal results, good genital hygiene was important to avoid infection, and constant lubrication of the necrotic tissue allowed for its easy removal (Fig. 5.8).

There are many similar clamps with different names, such as Ali's clamp, Tara KLamp, Solehring, etc., with various sizes depending on the diameter of the inner tube. Number 10 and 12 clamps are usually used for newborn and infant circumcisions, and number 14—20 clamps for older children. It is applied after sterile cleaning of the penis and administering local infiltrative anaesthesia. The plastic apparatus was removed between 24 h and 5 days depending on the age of the child. Children were called for routine follow-up visits 1 week and 1 month after removal of the clamp.

This sort of MC is usually called by some authors as a minimally invasive technique in comparison to the conventional surgical techniques, and many studies claim that utilizing such plastic clamps significantly reduces the complication rates, providing better cosmetic appearance than the conventional circumcisions, and they suggested it as the circumcision procedure of choice.[5]

ZHENXI RINGS

The prepuce is freed from and retracted over the glans. A grooved sleeve is passed over the glans to sit just behind the corona. The prepuce is then replaced over this sleeve. A hinged plastic clamping ring is fitted over the sleeve, the position of the prepuce is adjusted and the nut is tightened to hold the prepuce in place. An elastic cord is then wound tightly around the phallus, compressing the prepuce into the groove of the sleeve below it. This constricts the prepuce distally. The glans and frenulum are protected so that the frenulum remains intact. Too tight a sleeve can result in glans necrosis and too loose a sleeve can result in poor cosmetic outcome.

PREPEX DEVICE

This device is unique because of its use in adult MC without the need for anaesthesia (Fig. 5.9). It consists of a placement ring, an inner ring and an elastic ring. The placement ring is a carrier for the elastic ring to facilitate the application of the latter during the procedure. The inner ring has a groove on it for the lodgement of the elastic ring. When the device is applied, the prepuce is sandwiched between the inner ring and the elastic ring. The result is ischaemic necrosis of the 'trapped'

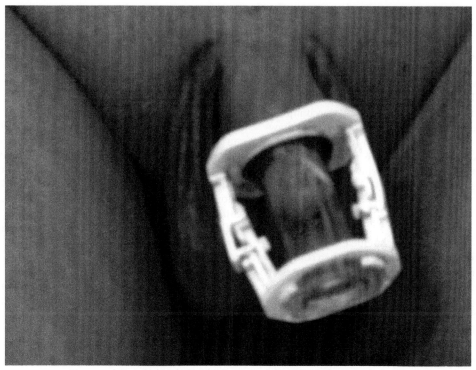

FIG. 5.8 Smart Klamp just before removal.

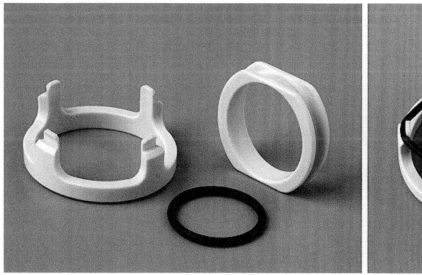
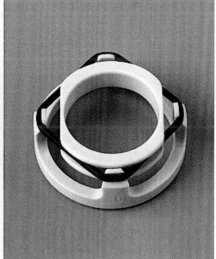

FIG. 5.9 PrePex device.

prepuce. The PrePex device is disassembled at about a week after placement and the withered prepuce is bloodlessly severed from the penis.[6]

The Chinese Shang Ring was recently introduced worldwide, and some authors claim that the use of this device is associated with a shorter operative time, lower blood loss volume and fewer postoperative complications than those in conventional MC techniques.[7] However, the use of Shang Ring also has some drawbacks: more time is required for wound healing, patients must endure pain for 7—16 days until the ring can be removed and wound dehiscence is relatively common after the ring removal.

THERMAL CUTTING

The thermocautery-assisted technique exploits the heat energy used for cauterizing (Fig. 5.10). When compared with the monopolar cautery technique, which uses an electrical current, the thermocautery-assisted method carries the heat locally. In the most recently developed thermocautery devices, the heat levels are adjustable according to the skin features of the patient. Previous studies have shown that optimum haemostasis is achieved with a temperature ranging between 100°C and 400°C. Although a range between 350°C and 900°C can be obtained within in vivo environments, the highest heat level is reduced by half in a bloody environment. It has been shown that the thermocautery technique results in similar wound healing when compared with the scalpel technique.[8]

Arslan et al.[9] performed mass circumcisions with thermocautery devices in Sudan, and they reported a complication rate of 0.086% in the early postsurgical period (3 weeks).

Many thermal injuries that result in either skin or penile loss will be discussed in Chapters 10 and 12.

SLEEVE RESECTION (DOUBLE CIRCULAR INCISION)

The foreskin is slid back along the shaft and a freehand cut is made around the shaft at the coronal sulcus by a scalpel (Figs. 5.11 and 5.12). The foreskin is returned to cover the glans and another cut is made around the shaft at the same position along its length as the first. A longitudinal cut is made between the two circumferential ones and the strip of skin is removed. The edges of the penile skin and preputial remnant are then pulled together and sutured. The glans and frenulum are not protected during the procedure. The frenulum can be included in the main cutting, cut separately or left intact. Results depend very much on the skill of the surgeon, but can be as tight or loose as desired with the scar line anywhere that is wanted. This technique is most commonly used in adults when circumcision is performed by a trained urologist (Video 5.1).

Stitching of the penile skin with remnant inner preputial layer should be achieved with meticulous undyed rapidly absorbable sutures, as persistent stitch marks and stitch sinus could be considered by children and parents as unaesthetic circumcision scar. Infection supervening the rough stitch material is not a rare complication, and this leads some surgeons to use different types of tissue glues and histoacryl to substitute penile skin stitching after MC. Furthermore, complications

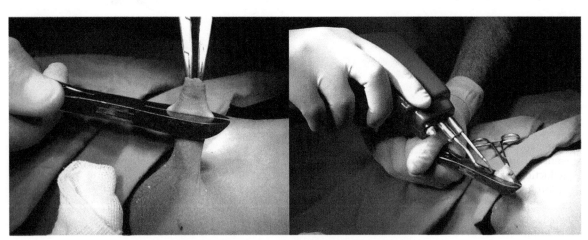

FIG. 5.10 Thermal cutting for guillotine circumcision.

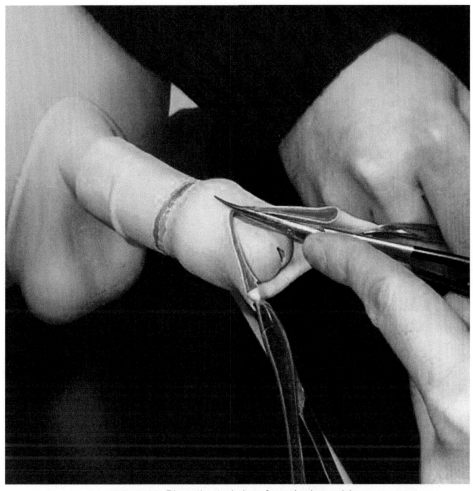

FIG. 5.11 Dissection technique for male circumcision.

that are specifically related to the suturing materials (e.g. granulomas, suture sinuses and/or marks) can negatively affect the cosmetic results, and will be discussed in Chapters 10 and 11.

The use of octyl cyanoacrylate (glue) in circumcision wound closure has been reported, and systematic reviews and meta-analyses provide the current best evidence, suggesting that the use of tissue glue for paediatric circumcision might be a valid alternative to the standard suture technique, with a clear benefit in the reduction of postoperative bleeding/haematoma formation and operating time, regardless of the technique used. Possible further benefits highlighted from systematic reviews include reduction in postoperative pain, improved cosmetic appearance and cost reduction.[10]

I prefer the method of double circular incision and stitching the edges of the skin with interrupted absorbable 6/0 stitches, even in neonates, as it will give an aesthetic tidy scar (Fig. 5.12).

With the recent attention to preserve the frenulum to avoid the consequent complication of meatal stenosis and to preserve the potential sensation of this structure, I started to preserve it during dissection and after completion of the procedure with two or more stitches applied to the frenular edges (Fig. 5.13, Video 5.2)

GUILLOTINE CIRCUMCISION

In Egypt and in most Middle East as well as many African countries, the most commonly used technique for MC is the bone cutting clamping, which crushes the

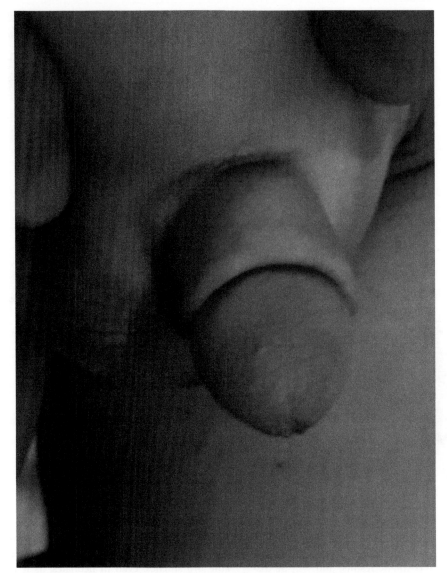

FIG. 5.12 A tidy circumcision scar, 3 months after the double circular incision technique.

preputial skin protecting the glans and gives a sharp skin cut, with a reasonable haemostasis. This method is used mainly in neonates and infants with a local anaesthetic (Fig. 5.14).

CIRCUMCISION STAPLER

A stapler with titanium staples is in use in many Asian countries, especially for adolescents (Fig. 5.15).

LASER CIRCUMCISION

Bleeding control and aesthetic skin edges could be obtained by using different laser beams to cut the prepuce; even better, gentle tissue dissection with simultaneous haemostasis was achieved by using an ultrasound dissection scalpel for circumcision (Fig. 5.16). Carbon dioxide laser was introduced in 1989 to excise the prepuce and weld its cut edges together, thus providing a completely bloodless operation. Suturing is optional,

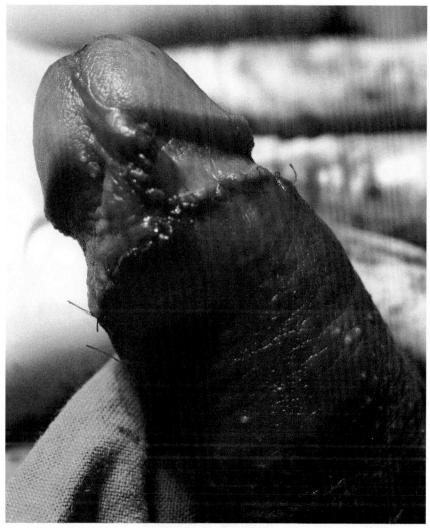

FIG. 5.13 Frenular preservation during the dissection method of circumcision.

as the laser can also be used to unite the cut edges. The technique allows exact proportions of skin and mucous membrane which will be removed. This method has been used by Joseph and Yap[11] in a total of 1154 patients ranging in age from infancy to 10 years. The neodymium:yttrium-aluminum-garnet (Nd:YAG) laser contact technique is also an effective laser-assisted procedure that is an alternative to the conventional technique in circumcision, with virtually no significant postoperative morbidity.[12]

Being a very common surgical procedure, circumcision demands careful selection of the operative procedure because different clamping and shielding methods are superior in terms of postoperative infection, whereas the open surgical method is better in terms of cosmeses and postoperative bleeding.

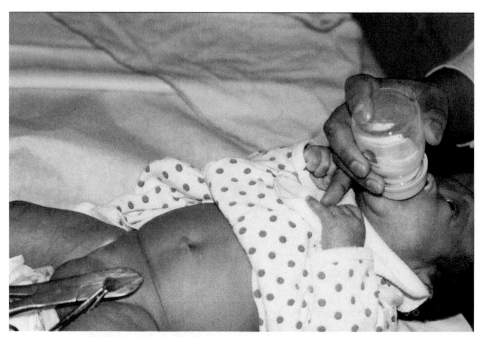

FIG. 5.14 Bone cutting guillotine technique, under local anesthesia.

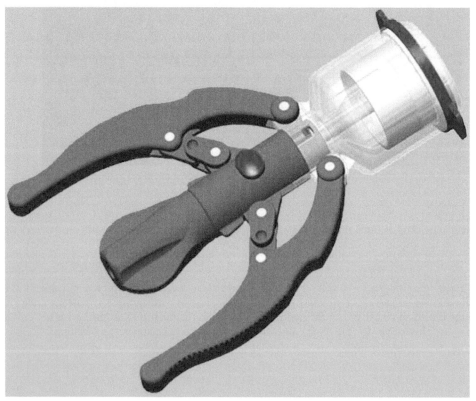

FIG. 5.15 Circumcision stapler.

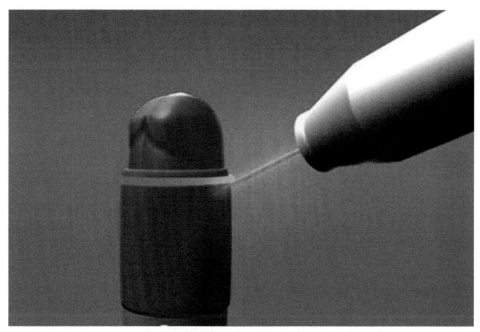

FIG. 5.16 Laser circumcision.

SUPPLEMENTARY DATA

Supplementary data related to this article can be found online at https://doi.org/10.1016/B978-0-323-68127-8.00005-3.

REFERENCES

1. http://www.circlist.com/instrstechs/who-manual-2008.pdf.
2. Bailey RC, Nyaboke I, Otieno FO. What device would be best for early infant male circumcision in East and Southern Africa? provider experiences and opinions with three different devices in Kenya. *PLoS One.* 2017;12:e0171445. https://doi.org/10.1371/journal.pone.0171445.
3. Wan J. Gomco circumcision clamp; an enduring and unexpected success. *Urology.* 2002;59(5):790–794. https://doi.org/10.1016/s0090-4295(01)01320-6. PMID 11992930.
4. Thornton J. A randomized trial of Mogen clamp versus Plastibell for neonatal male circumcision in Botswana. *J Acquir Immune Defic Syndr.* 2013;64(2):e12–e13.
5. Senel FM, Demirelli M, Oztek S. Minimally invasive circumcision with a novel plastic clamp technique: a review of 7,500 cases. *Pediatr Surg Int.* 2010;26:739–745. https://doi.org/10.1007/s00383-010-2632-3.
6. Abdulwahab-Ahmed A, Mungadi A. Techniques of male circumcision. *J Surg Tech Case Rep.* 2013;5(1):1–7. https://doi.org/10.4103/2006-8808.118588.
7. Awori QD, Lee RK, Li PS, et al. Surgical outcomes of newly trained Shang Ring circumcision providers. *J Acquir Immune Defic Syndr.* 2016;72(Suppl 1):S13–S17.
8. Tuncer AA, Bozkurt MF, Bayraktaroğlu A, et al. Examination of histopathological changes of scalpel, monopolar, bipolar, and thermocautery applications in rat experimental circumcision model. *Am J Transl Res.* 2017;9: 2306–2313.
9. Arslan D, Kalkan M, Yazgan H, Unuvar U, Şahin C. Collective circumcision performed in Sudan: evaluation in terms of early complications and alternative practice. *Urology.* 2013;81:864–868.
10. Martin A, Ramesh N, Kimber C, Pacilli M. The use of tissue glue for circumcision in children: systematic review and meta-analysis. *Urology.* 2018;115:21–28. https://doi.org/10.1016/j.urology.2018.01.022.
11. Joseph VT, Yap TL. Laser circumcision, a novel technique for day-care surgery. *Pediatr Surg Int.* 1995;10:434. https://doi.org/10.1007/BF00182253.
12. How A, Ong C, Jacobsen A, et al. Carbon dioxide laser circumcisions for children. *Pediatr Surg Int.* 2003;19:11. https://doi.org/10.1007/s00383-002-0894-0.

Anaesthesia and Analgesia for Male Circumcision and Its Complications

MOHAMED A BAKY FAHMY, MD, FRCS

ABSTRACT

There is considerable evidence that newborns who are circumcised without analgesia experience pain and physiologic stress. Neonatal physiologic responses to circumcision pain include changes in heart rate, blood pressure, oxygen saturation and cortisol levels. One report has noted that circumcised infants exhibit a stronger pain response to subsequent routine immunization than do uncircumcised infants.

KEYWORDS

Dorsal penile nerve block; Subcutaneous ring block; Topical anaesthesia.

RELEVANT ANATOMY

The penis is composed of the paired corpora cavernosa and the corpus spongiosum. The proximal portion of the corpus spongiosum is referred to as the bulb of the penis and the glans represents its distal expansion. The urethra traverses the corpus spongiosum to exit at the meatus. The fascial layers of the penis are continuous with the fascial layers of the perineum and lower abdomen. Dartos fascia represents the superficial penile fascia. Deep to this lies the Buck fascia, which covers the tunica albuginea of the penile bodies. Proximally, the Buck fascia is in continuity with the suspensory ligament of the penis, which attaches to the symphysis pubis (Fig. 6.1).

The penis is supplied by a superficial system of arteries that arise from the external pudendal arteries and a deep system of arteries that stem from the internal pudendal arteries. The superficial blood supply lies in the superficial penile fascia and supplies the penile skin and prepuce. The internal pudendal artery, which arises from the hypogastric artery, gives rise to the penile artery, which then gives rise to the bulbourethral artery, the urethral artery and the cavernous artery (deep artery of the penis) before terminating as the dorsal artery of the penis.

NERVOUS SUPPLY OF THE PENIS AND PREPUCE

Penile innervation is via both autonomic (parasympathetic and sympathetic) and somatic (motor and sensory) pathways. Erection and detumescence are largely regulated via the autonomic system. Sympathetic and parasympathetic nerves coalesce to form the cavernous nerve, which penetrates the corpora cavernosa to exert its effect on erection. Sensation and contraction of penile musculature occurs via the somatic nerves.

AUTONOMIC INNERVATION

Between the T11 and L2 spinal segments, the sympathetic trunk begins and its fibres then form the sympathetic chain ganglia, which continue caudally to the inferior mesenteric and superior hypogastric plexuses. Further sympathetic fibres exit to form the hypogastric nerves and ultimately the sympathetic portions of the pelvic plexus.

Between the S2-S4 spinal cord segments, the parasympathetic pathway originates and its fibres also continue caudally to the pelvic plexus (Fig. 6.2), where they join the aforementioned sympathetic nerves. Together, these nerves then join to form a network of nervous tissue that passes along the lateral and posterior aspects of the prostate to create the cavernous nerves. Stimulation of the sympathetic trunk via the cavernous nerves results in detumescence.

SOMATIC INNERVATION

Sensory receptors in the penile skin and glans are unique to the human body. They are composed of free nerve endings comprising unmyelinated C fibres and thin myelinated A delta fibres. These coalesce into the dorsal

Complications in Male Circumcision. https://doi.org/10.1016/B978-0-323-68127-8.00006-5

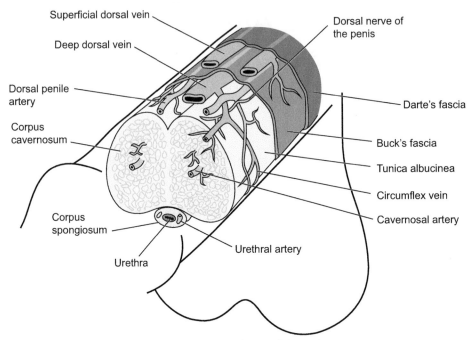

FIG. 6.1 Anatomic layers of the penis.

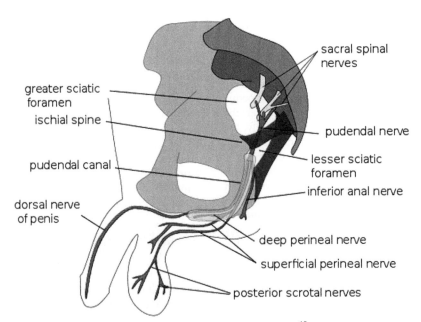

FIG. 6.2 Nervous system of the penis.[10]

nerve of the penis, which ultimately forms the pudendal nerve. The pudendal nerve then enters the S2-S4 nerve roots at the spinal cord. Via the spinothalamic and spinoreticular pathways, sensations such as touch, pain and temperature are perceived (Fig. 6.2).

Somatic nerve supply to the penis comes by way of the pudendal nerves, which eventually produce the dorsal nerves of the penis on each side. Although cutaneous innervation to the penis is primarily from branches of the pudendal nerve, the proximal portion is supplied by the ilioinguinal nerve after it leaves the superficial inguinal ring. The prepuce has somatosensory innervation by the dorsal nerve of the penis and branches of the perineal nerve. The glans is primarily innervated by free nerve endings and has poor fine-touch discrimination.[1]

GENERAL ANAESTHESIA

General recommendations in most centres in the United States indicate the use of a general anesthetic for children aged 4 months and older for circumcision and this may carry a small risk. Studies have stated that dormicum, propofol and ketamine are commonly used for sedoanalgesia of children undergoing male circumcision (MC). The combination of midazolam and ketamine (11.7%) was chosen most frequently, and this is may provide a better hemodynamic stability for surgical conditions. It is thus surprising that only 71% of paediatricians, 56% of family practitioners and only 25% of obstetricians in the United States use analgesia and anaesthesia for MC.[2]

REGIONAL ANAESTHESIA

Children undergoing MC are ideal candidates for different types of outpatient regional anaesthesia. Success is mainly dependent on good organization, including careful selection of the patient, professional and skilled anaesthetic care and the proper knowledge for avoiding postoperative problems. Anaesthesiologists frequently choose laryngeal mask and the regional anaesthesia method of caudal block with bupivacaine and levobupivacaine for circumcision operations. In the recent years, the use of ultrasound has become popular in performing regional anaesthesia, with an increasing number of anaesthesiologists using these techniques in their daily clinical practice.

LOCAL ANAESTHESIA
Dorsal Penile Nerve Block

Dorsal penile nerve block (DPNB) was firstly described by Bateman in 1975, and since then, it has gained increasing popularity because of the ease of performance and perceived safety. It has an estimated complication rate of 0.18%.[3]

DPNB represents 85% of anaesthetic use in the United States and is effective, even in low-birth-weight infants. It involves injection of a local anaesthetic at the 10- and 2-o'clock positions at the base of the penis, where the dorsal penile nerve is situated.[4] (Figs. 6.3 and 6.4).

DPNB is very effective in reducing the behavioural and physiologic indicators of pain caused by circumcision. Compared with control subjects who received no analgesia, neonates with DPNB cry 45%−76% less, have 34%−50% smaller increases in heart rate and have smaller decreases in oxygen saturation during the procedure. Additionally, DPNB lidocaine attenuates the adrenocortical stress response compared with control subjects who received no injections or injections of saline. The technique of Kirya and Werthmann[5] is used most commonly to perform the block, in which a 27-gauge needle is used to inject 0.4 mL of 1% lidocaine, to be administered at both the 10- and 2-o'clock positions at the base of the penis. The needle is directed posteromedially 3−5 mm on each side until it enters Buck fascia. After aspiration, the local anaesthetic is injected. Systemic lidocaine levels obtained by using this technique demonstrated peak concentrations at 60 min, well below toxic ranges. Several studies evaluating the efficacy of DPNB reported bruising as the most frequent complication. Haematomas were rarely seen and caused no long-term injury; a single report of penile necrosis may have been secondary to the surgical technique rather than to the DPNB.[6] (Video 6.1).

Subcutaneous Ring Block

In a study, a subcutaneous circumferential ring of 0.8 mL of 1% lidocaine without epinephrine at the mid-shaft of the penis, which had initially been used for post-circumcision analgesia, is simpler and was found to be more effective than eutectic mixture of local anaesthetics (EMLA, a eutectic mixture of lidocaine and prilocaine) cream (AstraZeneca, Wilmington, DE, USA) or DPNB.[6] Pain from the infiltration of a local anaesthetic is short-lived and significantly less than the pain from an unanaesthetized circumcision.

Although all treatment groups experienced an attenuated pain response, the ring block (RB) appeared to prevent crying and increases in heart rate more consistently than did EMLA cream or DPNB throughout all stages of circumcision. In another study, after a subcutaneous injection of lidocaine had been given at the level of the corona, it was noted that fewer infants cried during the dissection of the foreskin, placement of the bell and clamping of the Gomco when compared with those infants with a DPNB. Additionally, the cortisol

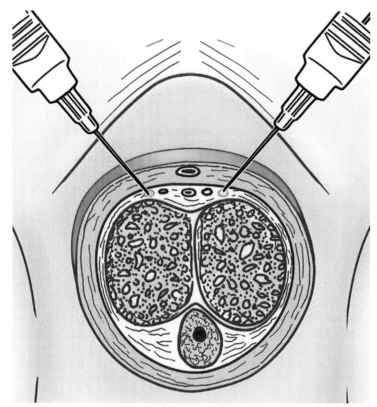

FIG. 6.3 Pictorial representation of dorsal nerve block at 10- and 2-o'clock sites around the dorsal nerves of the penis.

response was diminished in the subcutaneous group when compared with the DPNB group. No complications have been reported in this simple and highly effective technique (Figs. 6.5 and 6.6).

We found that the combination of dorsal nerve block and subcutaneous ring anaesthesia is very effective and has minimal adverse effects in all age groups of children undergoing MC by either the guillotine or dissection method of MC (Video 6.2).

TOPICAL ANAESTHESIA

Routine neonatal circumcision is commonly performed under topical anaesthesia with EMLA cream, which is usually applied with polyethylene sheet closure one hour before the procedure (Fig. 6.7).

Dermal analgesia is achieved within 1 h after application and occlusion, with a maximal effect at 2–3 h and influence lingering on for 1–2 h after removal. In children, the recommended EMLA dosing depends on age and body weight.[4]

Immediate hypersensitivity reactions have rarely been reported with local anaesthetics; however, delayed type hypersensitivity (type IV) reactions have been more commonly reported and benzocaine appears to be the most common culprit.

Type IV reactions to EMLA have been shown to occur because of both its constituents, and even contact urticaria has been described in some babies. Adverse effects related to the use of EMLA are mild reactions such as oedema, erythema and transient pallor, late hyperpigmentation and contact dermatitis, both allergic and irritant, have been reported. Rare nonallergic reactions, such as purpura formation, may occur probably via a direct toxic effect.

Methaemoglobinemia and seizures are serious reported complications because a metabolite of prilocaine can oxidize haemoglobin to methaemoglobin. When measured, blood levels of methaemoglobin in neonates after the application of 1 g of EMLA cream have been well below toxic levels.[7]

(A)

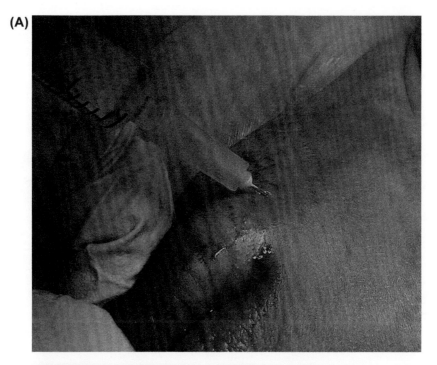

(B)

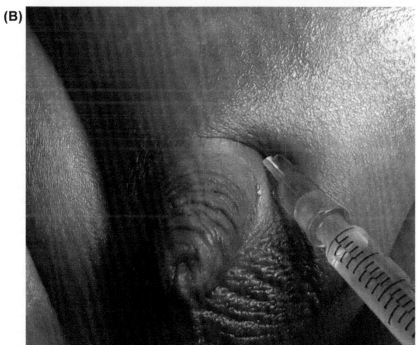

FIG. 6.4 Dorsal nerve block; **(A)** injection at 10 o'clock. **(B)** injection at 2-o'clock sites around the dorsal nerves of the penis.

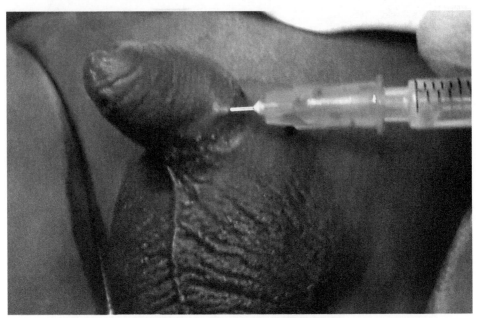

FIG. 6.5 Subcutaneous ring block.

RECOMMENDATIONS OF ANAESTHESIA AND ANALGESIA FOR MALE CIRCUMCISION

1. Paracetamol is frequently used for postoperative analgesia after circumcision.
2. A DPNB with an RB, using proper technique, is the most effective technique to provide anaesthesia during neonatal circumcision (Level 1-2 evidence, Grade A recommendation).
3. Topical local anaesthetics alone are inferior to nerve and RBs and require an adequate time interval for efficacy and can be used as an adjunct to penile blocks (Level 1−2 evidence, Grade A recommendation).
4. Oral sucrose, non-nutritive sucking, music and other environmental interventions should only be used as an adjunct to these methods (Level 1−3 evidence, Grade A recommendation).
   - A double-blinded randomized controlled trial compared three combination analgesics used during circumcision (EMLA + sucrose, EMLA + sucrose + DPNB and EMLA + sucrose + RB) with the traditional topical analgesic EMLA cream alone and found that during neonatal circumcision in boys, the most effective analgesia is RB combined with oral sucrose and EMLA cream.[8]
   - Pacifiers, especially with glucose or sucrose, are also effective (pain score is 1 as opposed to 7 with placebo). A milk formula could also be given to the baby during the procedure, and it is our practice to give it even for the babies who received dorsal nerve block or ring anaesthesia (Fig. 6.8).
   - There is considerable evidence that newborns who are circumcised without analgesia experience pain and physiologic stress. Neonatal physiologic responses to circumcision pain include changes in heart rate, blood pressure, oxygen saturation and cortisol levels. One report has noted that circumcised infants exhibit a stronger pain response to subsequent routine immunization than do uncircumcised infants.[9] Several methods to provide analgesia for circumcision have been evaluated. There is a need to develop standard anaesthesia protocols within the frame of international recommendations for circumcision, which is the most commonly performed outpatient surgical procedure (Fig. 6.9).

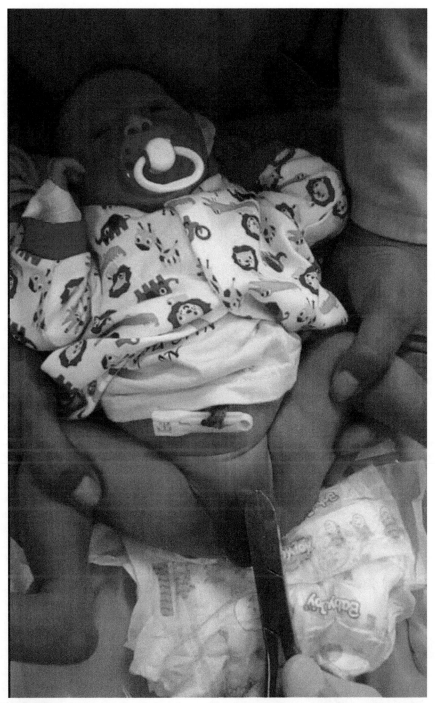

FIG. 6.6 A baby completely calm during circumcision by guillotine method after both dorsal nerve and subcutaneous ring blocks.

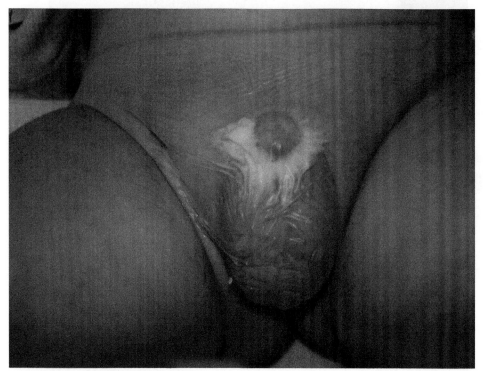

FIG. 6.7 EMLA (eutectic mixture of local anaesthetics) cream applied over the penis with a polyethylene sheet.

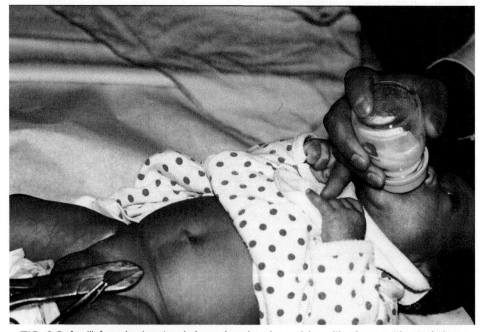

FIG. 6.8 A milk formula given to a baby undergoing circumcision with a bone cutting technique.

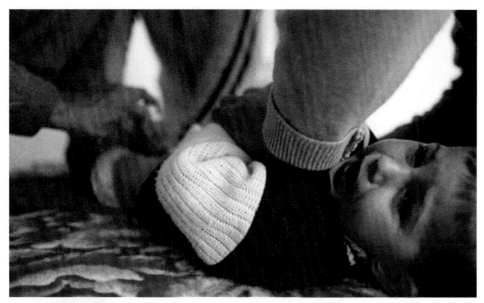

FIG. 6.9 An apprehensive child undergoing a ritual circumcision in a rural area.

SUPPLEMENTARY DATA

Supplementary data related to this article can be found online at https://doi.org/10.1016/B978-0-323-68127-8.00006-5.

REFERENCES

1. Hsu GL, Hsieh CH, Wen HS, Hsu WL, Chen CW. Anatomy of the human penis: the relationship of the architecture between skeletal and smooth muscles. *J Androl*. 2004;25:426–431.
2. Ozkan A, Okur M, Kaya M, et al. Sedoanalgesia in pediatric daily surgery. *Int J Clin Exp Med*. 2013;6(7):576–582 ([PubMed]).
3. Bateman DV. Correspondence. *Anaesthesia*. 1975;30:101.
4. Brady-Fryer B, Wiebe N, Lander JA. Pain relief for neonatal circumcision. *Cochrane Database Syst Rev*. 2004;4. CD004217.
5. Kirya C, Werthmann Jr MW. Neonatal circumcision and penile dorsal nerve block—a painless procedure. *J Pediatr*. 1978;92:998–1000.
6. Nossaman VE, Nossaman BD. Regional anesthetic techniques for the pediatric patient. In: Kaye A, Urman R, Vadivelu N, eds. *Essentials of Regional Anesthesia*. Cham: Springer; 2018. https://doi.org/10.1007/978-3-319-74838-2_15.
7. Capron F, Perry D, Capolaghi B. Convulsive crisis and methemoglobinemia after the application of anesthetic cream. *Arch Pediatr*. 1998;5(7):812. [Pubmed].
8. Sharara-Chami R, Lakissian Z, Charafeddine L, Milad N, El-Hout Y. Combination analgesia for neonatal circumcision: a randomized controlled trial. *Pediatrics*. Nov 2017:e20171935. https://doi.org/10.1542/peds.2017-1935.
9. Holve RL, Bronberger PJ, Groveman HD. Regional anesthesia during newborn circumcision: effect on infant pain response. *Clin Pediatr*. 1983;22:813–818. [Medline].
10. Häggström M. Medical gallery of Mikael Häggström 2014. *WikiJournal of Medicine*. 2014;1(2). https://doi.org/10.15347/wjm/2014.008. ISSN 2002-4436.

CHAPTER 7

Prevalence of Male Circumcision Complications

MOHAMED A BAKY FAHMY, MD, FRCS

ABSTRACT

As with any surgical procedure, circumcision can result in complications, and the most common early (intra-operative) complications tend to be minor and treatable, such as minor bleeding, swelling. However, serious complications may occur during or immediately after the procedure, including death from excess bleeding, severe urethral injuries and complete or partial amputation of the entire penis or the glans. Late postoperative complications include formation of a skin bridge between the penile shaft and the glans, infection, urinary retention, meatal ulcer, fistulas and other rare complications. Loss of penile sensitivity, sexual dysfunction and psychic impaction are considered as remote complications by some authors. Prevalence of reported complications of male circumcision ranged from 0% to 50.1%, and late complications of 7.39% prevalence were reported.

KEYWORDS

Classifications; Concealed penis; Immunocompromised; Megameatus intact prepuce; Obesity; Scrotal transposition.

As with any surgical procedure, circumcision can result in complications, and the most common early (intra-operative) complications tend to be minor and treatable, such as minor bleeding, swelling. However, serious complications may occur during or immediately after the procedure, including death from excess bleeding, severe urethral injuries and complete or partial amputation of the entire penis or the glans. A retrospective analysis of all infants who underwent circumcision from 2001 to 2010 in an inpatient hospital during the first 30 days of life (Nationwide Inpatient Sample) reported 200 early deaths among 9,833,110 infants (1 death per 49,166 circumcisions), with associated comorbid conditions such as cardiac disease, coagulopathy, fluid and electrolyte disorders and pulmonary circulatory disorders.[1]

Late postoperative complications include formation of a skin bridge between the penile shaft and the glans, infection, urinary retention, meatal ulcer, fistulas and other rare complications. Loss of penile sensitivity, sexual dysfunction and psychic impaction are considered as remote complications by some authors. Prevalence of reported complications of male circumcision (MC) ranged from 0% to 50.1%, and late complications of 7.39% prevalence were reported.[2]

A systematic review on complications of neonatal and infant circumcisions estimated a complication rate from 0% to 16% (median 2%) in 16 prospective studies.[3] Circumcisions performed in older children were associated with more complications (median 6%) when compared with those carried out in neonates and infants. A systematic review on safety and efficacy of nontherapeutic MC in 5228 men (aged 15–49 years) showed a 4.8% incidence of complications. The most common complication was postoperative infection (1.5%), followed by bleeding (1.3%). Complication rates in the three HIV trials conducted in Africa ranged between 1.7% and 8%.[4]

In 2010, a review of literature found that MC performed by medical providers have a typical complication rate of 1.5% for babies and 6% for older children, with a few cases of severe complications.[5] In Africa and the developing countries, the circumcision rate was 87%, with a higher rate of complications reaching 20.2%.

According to Pieretti et al.,[6] almost 5% of paediatric cases performed at a tertiary institution in the United States over a 5-year span, with an estimated cost of $685,608, were related to complications of newborn circumcision.

The literature review by the American Academy of Pediatrics (AAP) and a large detailed study by the Centers for Disease Control and Prevention (CDC) of 1.4 million MCs performed from 2001 to 10 (93% in newborns) have determined that adverse events from MC occur in less than 0.5% of newborns and almost all are minor and immediately treatable with complete resolution. In the CDC study, serious adverse events arising from early infant MC were extremely rare (1 penile stricture, penile replantations, 16 cases of artery suture and 3 partial, but no complete, penile amputations).[7]

FACTORS AFFECTING CIRCUMCISION COMPLICATION RATE

Factors Related to the Age at Which Circumcision is Done

The timing of surgery can be predictive of complications, as bleeding-related complications are higher in older infants. Penile adhesions and secondary buried penis are more likely in infants with a higher weight for length percentile. It is usually reported that the rate of complications is higher among adults than in neonates undergoing MC. I think this a false impression because most of the adult cases were circumcised in hospitals or specialized centers, so the complications are recordable and traceable, but for neonates, most cases were usually circumcised in a remote area away from detection of complications and most cases are not strictly followed up for a sufficient time to pick up complications; therefore, in my opinion, the rate of complications is higher in neonates than what is reported in most literature.

The prospective studies in older boys also found virtually no serious adverse events but a higher frequency of complications (up to 14%), even when conducted by trained providers in sterile settings.[8] The lower frequency of complications among neonates and infants is likely to be attributable to the simpler nature of the procedure in this age group and to the healing capability of the newborn. This advantage is illustrated by the US study in which no complications were observed among 98 boys circumcised in the first month of life, but 30% of boys aged 3–8.5 months had significant postoperative bleeding. There are alternatives to suturing, such as use of disposable clamps or cyanoacrylate glue, and further research in this area is needed.[9]

Three studies reported substantial variation in complication frequencies by age or circumcision method. For example, a US study of circumcision by the Gomco clamp stratified by age at circumcision found no complications in 98 boys circumcised neonatally but reported that 12/32 (30%) infants aged 3–8.5 months had postoperative bleeding requiring suture repair.[8]

These 32 boys were circumcised under general anaesthesia, and no complications from the anaesthesia were reported.

In another study, complications were seen more frequently using the Plastibell technique (12/381; 3.1%) than the sleeve technique (4/205; 1.95%).[10]

FACTORS RELATED TO THE HEALTH STATUS OF THE BABY TO BE CIRCUMCISED

- Hemorrhagic and infectious complications are higher among babies who are premature, have jaundice and have coagulopathy such as sickle cell disease and haemophilia. Children with blood dyscrasia can undergo circumcision under appropriate treatment and care.[11]
- Immunocompromised and diabetic babies and babies with hidden septic focus may be vulnerable for secondary infection if circumcised early in life. In such cases, local genital infection after circumcision may be disseminated, leading to septicaemia and other rarely reported cases of meningitis.
- Obesity, in general, and excessive suprapubic fat, in particular, have a worse effect in MC, with an increased incidence of post-circumcision bleeding as an early complication and penile adhesions with a hidden penis as late complication.[12] An increased weight for length percentile in male infants before and after circumcision may be significantly associated with webbed and hidden penis. So it is advisable to postpone MC in overweight children if there is a chance for weight reduction; otherwise special precautions should be taken, such as proper haemostasis, meticulous suturing of the circumcised edges and proper follow-up (Fig 7.1).

CIRCUMCISING AN ABNORMAL BABY OR A DEFORMED PENIS

Neonatal circumcision should be performed on medically stable, term infants without other medical conditions, which requires ongoing management or increased risk of surgery. Routine neonatal circumcision should not be carried out in children with congenital anomalies including the penis itself, the prepuce, urethra, scrotum or testicles; we encountered many cases circumcised at the neonatal age with a wide range of congenital anomalies either common anomalies such as hypospadias (Fig. 7.2), epispadias (Fig. 7.3), ventral curvature and chordee (Fig. 7.4), penoscrotal webbing (Fig. 7.5) or rare cases of penile rotation (Fig. 7.6), markedly concealed penis (CP) (Fig. 7.7) and babies with different grades of penoscrotal transposition (Fig. 7.8).

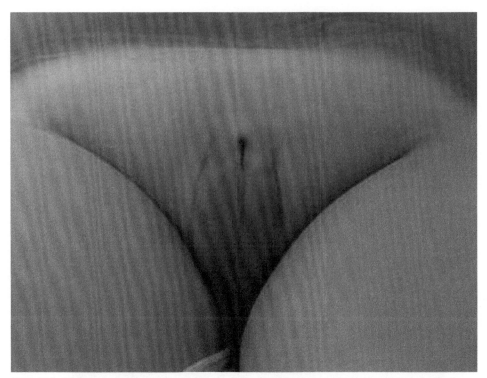

FIG. 7.1 Obesity, in general, and excessive suprapubic fat increase the incidence of complications.

Babies who had a webbed or a buried penis are more liable to several complications and usually end with an untidy scar. Cases of webbed penis are not uncommon, and if circumcision is performed without recognition, a most unsatisfactory appearance is created, with the penis buried in a tent-like fold of skin. Recircumcision to remove the excess skin makes the situation worse by drawing hair-bearing scrotal skin onto the penis without getting rid of the tent-like appearance (Fig. 7.5). Cases of aposthia and microposthia will end with severe penile complications if not recognized by an expert paediatric surgeon during ritual MC.

Many cases with different degrees of penile rotation are usually unrecognized during ritual circumcision or if they are circumcised by a gynaecologist early after they are born; such cases may stand later on as a medicolegal issue, as the family will accuse the circumciser attributing that the congenital anomaly was induced by MC. In some of these conditions, circumcision may lead to a disastrous outcome, or it may end with a hidden complication, which will not be obvious except at adolescence with the start of sexual activities. In such cases, MC could be performed with appropriate technical modifications, but this requires expert paediatric urologists or plastic surgeons.

Some children with a hypospadias variant termed megameatus intact prepuce hypospadias have a normal foreskin and a distal hypospadias that is only uncovered during a circumcision; MC in such cases may end in medicolegal problems (Fig. 7.9). Actually, most children with this variant or who had a distal hypospadias can proceed with a circumcision; however, this requires an ability to recognize the severity of the anomaly and therefore, as a general rule, all boys with hypospadias should ideally not undergo circumcision without consulting a paediatric urologist.

Also it is our recommendation to physicians and parents to postpone MC in babies who had a congenital hydrocele; in such cases, it is difficult to wrap the circumcised penis in bandage, with a high rate of post-circumcision bleeding and haematoma formation. Also, many cases may end with an incomplete circumcision or CP, caused by an incomplete preputial cut, and this eventually leads to an untidy scar and cicatricial phimosis. It is strange enough to see such babies undergoing repeated circumcision by inexperienced surgeons, creating more complications, mainly with deficient ventral skin (Fig. 7.10).

Babies with a congenital inguinal hernia and undescended testicle should have a priority for these

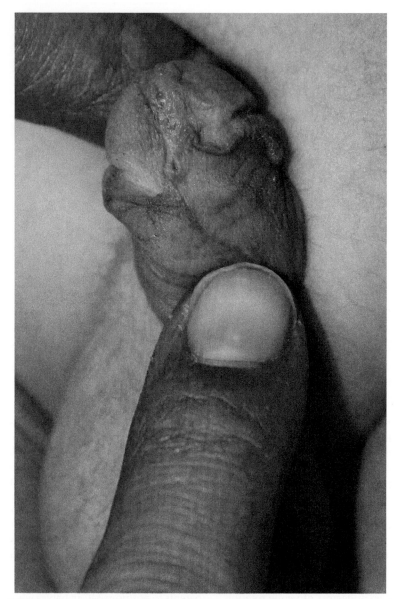

FIG. 7.2 A case of a coronal hypospadias circumcised early in the neonatal period.

conditions to be operated before undergoing MC; otherwise, circumcision could be carried on the same setting after completion of the primary surgery for the hernia and undescended testicle if the situation permits. It is a trend of many general surgeons to do MC along other procedures such as hernia repair, but sometimes the hernia surgery may pass through serious complications, while the baby had two procedures done, as in

baby seen in Fig 7.11, in whom the hernia repair was complicated by intestinal obstruction necessitating re-exploration and bowel resection.

In some rural areas, the paramedic personnel or even the physician, in response to the family wishes and pressure, may commit circumcision in a critically ill baby with a serious life-threatening congenital anomaly without a proper evaluation of the baby; it seems that

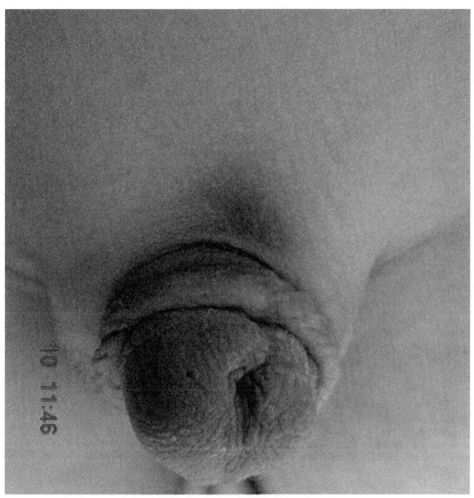

FIG. 7.3 A circumcised baby with epispadias.

the circumciser will do his/her job regardless of the condition of the penis or the general condition of the baby. Fig. 7.12 depicts a case of androgen insensitivity syndrome who came for sex assignment after puberty, but the circumcised small phallus can be recognized. In Fig. 7.13 a baby who had an imperforate anus, but circumcision was done for him immediately after delivery by the gynaecologist, without recognizing this obvious serious anomaly.

It is difficult to imagine how a penis with a serious penile malformation can pass through neonatal MC, for example, the patient in Fig. 7.14, who had a severe vascular malformation but was circumcised.

Thus the caveat must be 'do the right circumcision in the right patient using the correct surgical technique'.

CIRCUMCISION OF CONCEALED PENIS

Penis should be assessed carefully before performing circumcision in terms of 'how visible' or 'how concealed' it is, especially the professionals doing routine circumcision should be informed about the entity of CP and cautioned that they refer the suspicious cases to where patients can receive appropriate treatment. Circumcision itself might have contributed to the concealment in some cases (Fig. 7.15).

Some circumcision complications appear to be more frequent among cases with complete or partial CP. Especially the partial CP often remains unrecognized before circumcision and this leads to increased rates of cosmetic complications, such as glanular adhesions and secondary phimosis. Estimating the preoperative

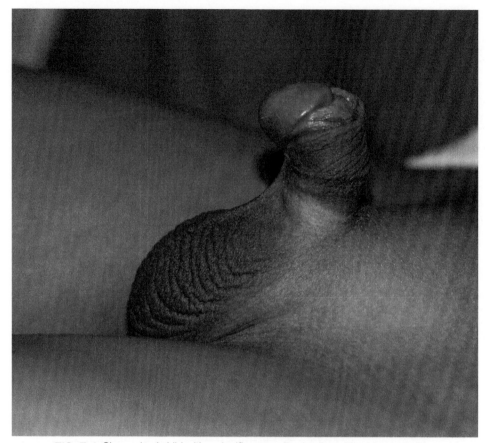

FIG. 7.4 Circumcised child with a significant penile chordee without hypospadias.

penile length may help predict the cosmetic outcome after circumcision, which in turn might alter the management. Sometimes the concealment is relative and is only due to the presence of a marked hernia or hydrocele, especially in bilateral cases, so it is wise to postpone MC in such cases (Fig. 7.16).

Penile visibility index calculation before circumcision might help predict some cosmetic complications beforehand and provide better information for the parents. Prospective studies are needed to corroborate our analysis.[13]

Proper examination of boys by a physician before undergoing circumcision provides a golden chance for the detection of penile anomalies, which can be corrected at the same session or later on, and the arrangements for performing circumcision in hospitals by the medical staff should be favored. The misleading perception of underestimation of the procedure when it is ritually performed should be corrected. Admission to a hospital for circumcision provides an opportunity to examine the genitalia of boys properly, but the most important goal is to change the public's perception of circumcision, who generally underestimate the procedure. They should be informed about all the complications and consequences in order to have their children operated in a hospital setting by the medical staff.[14]

FACTORS RELATED TO THE CIRCUMCISER

Circumcision by non-medically trained personnel usually followed by a high rate of both early and late complications; a high frequency of complications was seen in a retrospective study from Turkey of 407 boys circumcised at two traditional mass circumcision events.[15]

The complications were substantially more common when circumcision was performed freehand (27% excluding incomplete circumcision) than by using Plastibell (8%) or was performed by midwives (19%) than by doctors (7%). Interestingly, among circumcisions

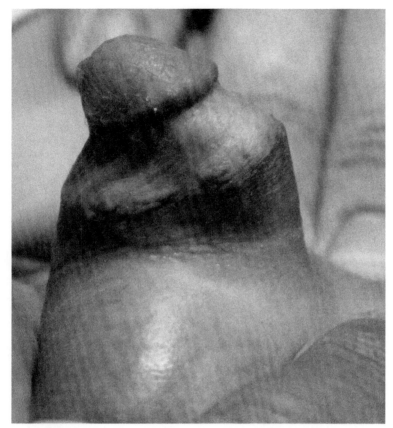

FIG. 7.5 A baby circumcised with a marked penoscrotal webbing.

performed by doctors, the frequency of complications at a university teaching hospital was 1.6% compared with 20% at private hospitals.

A study from Iran reported a late-phase complication frequency of 2.7% following traditional circumcision and a further 5% had excessive residual foreskin. This frequency was similar to that in circumcisions performed by urologists or surgeons (2.8%), but lower than that for general practitioners/paediatricians (6.1%) or paramedic personnel (9.1%).[16]

Current ongoing operator experience was shown to be an important factor in lower bleeding complication rate when compared with patient-related variables and long-term operator experience.

In most studies designed in a country or center that is trying to promote circumcision, the true frequency of complications are commonly underestimated.

Among doctors, the reported frequency of complications at a public university teaching hospital was 1.6% compared with 20% at private hospitals, where the level of training and supervision was lower. A much higher frequency (90%) was seen at the mission hospital, which acts as a referral centre for complicated circumcisions. The studies with the highest frequency of complications were in Pakistan and the United Kingdom. The study in Pakistan reported on 200 infants circumcised under local anaesthesia at a military hospital using either the freehand or the bone cutter method.[17]

In the UK study, 1129 infants were circumcised by nurses using the Plastibell under local anaesthesia, and overall 125 (11.1%) infants required some degree of follow-up, with complications seen in 5.5%. The most common complication involved the Plastibell ring device itself (3.6%).[18]

Finally, a Turkish study reports complications following a hospital-based mass circumcision exercise, in which 700 boys were circumcised over 5 days. Excluding the cases of bleeding stopped by simple compression, 8% of boys had a complication, most commonly infection (2.7%) and inadequate foreskin removal accompanied by secondary phimosis (2.1%).[19]

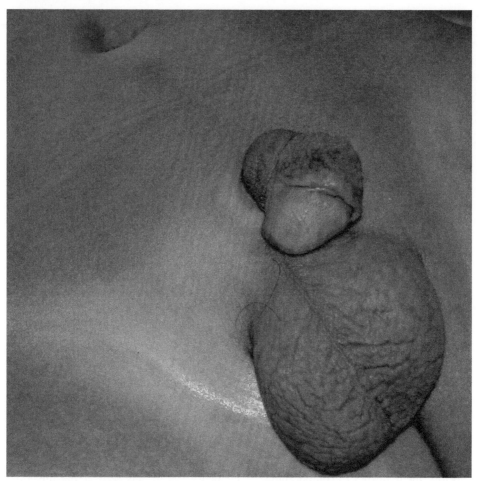

FIG. 7.6 A circumcised baby, while he had a significant right-side penile rotation.

FACTORS RELATED TO THE METHOD AND TECHNIQUE OF CIRCUMCISION

The results of varying techniques may also be a possible factor affecting complication rates. Results from a small randomized controlled trial that compared two surgical techniques (sleeve vs. Plastibell) in older children showed that late complications occurred in 12% of the cases that used the sleeve technique versus 5% with the Plastibell device.[20]

REPORTING OF THE RATE OF CIRCUMCISION COMPLICATIONS

The problem with MC complications is mainly due to improper or biased reporting, which may be due to inadequate follow-up or an intention to underestimate the complications in favour of promoting the safety of MC.

The basis in studies reporting the rate of Complications arise from the following:

- Circumcision is a common surgical procedure, but few epidemiologic studies have reported on the frequency of adverse events, which are most commonly bleeding and infection. Serious adverse events are rare, but there is a wide variation in the reported frequencies of such events.
- Limitations related to the design of the epidemiologic studies.
- Timing of surgery can be predictive of complications, such as bleeding-related complications, which are higher in older infants.
- Variable length of follow-up between, and within, studies that may affect the estimated frequency of complications.

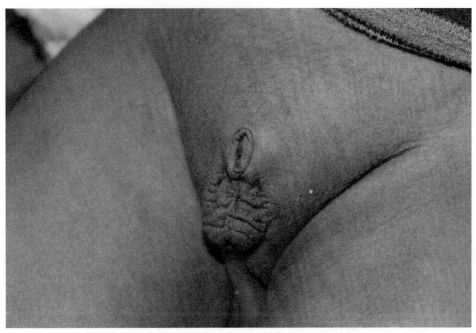

FIG. 7.7 A circumcised baby with a significant buried penis.

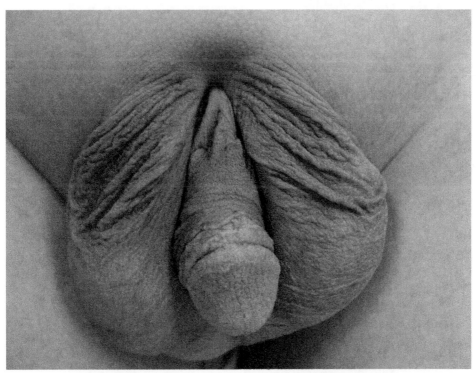

FIG. 7.8 A baby with scrotal transposition circumcised early in infancy.

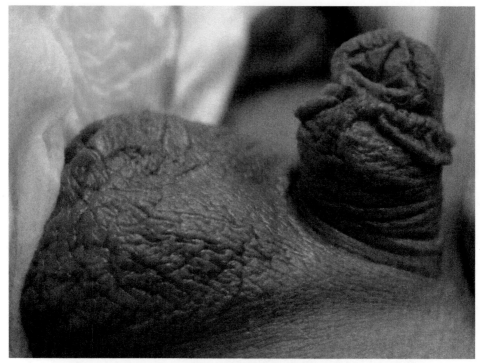

FIG. 7.9 A baby circumcised while he has a megameatus intact prepuce.

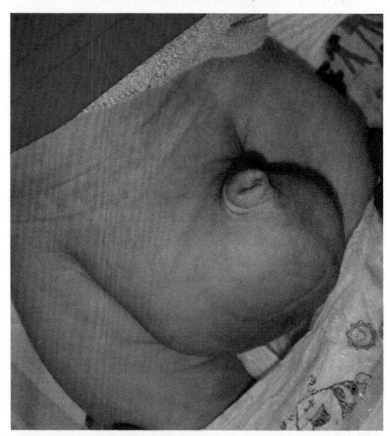

FIG. 7.10 An infant with a marked right-side hydrocele was circumcised early and developed an acquired phimosis with a concealed penis.

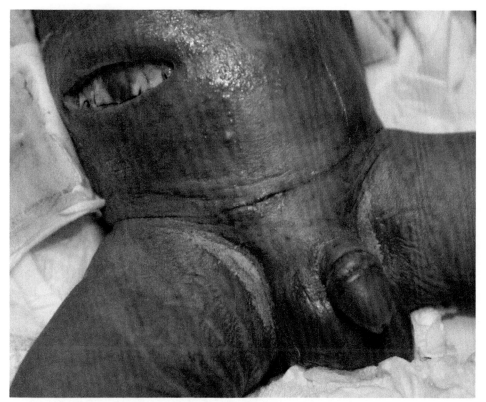

FIG. 7.11 A baby was circumcised during inguinal hernia surgery, and he developed an intestinal obstruction that required exploration later on.

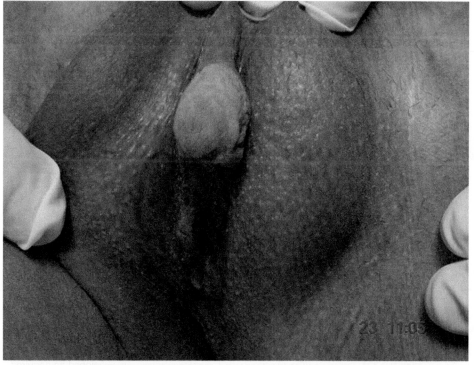

FIG. 7.12 An adolescent with androgen insensitivity syndrome, and he was circumcised during neonatal age.

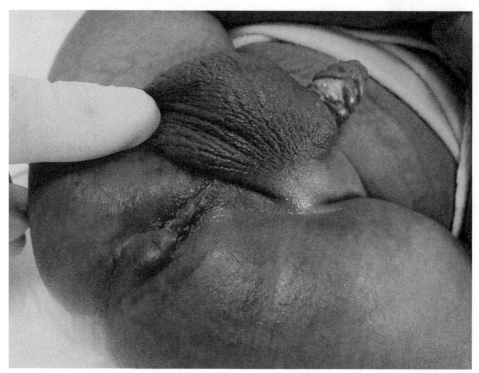

FIG. 7.13 A neonate with an imperforate anus circumcised without recognition of his obstructed bowel.

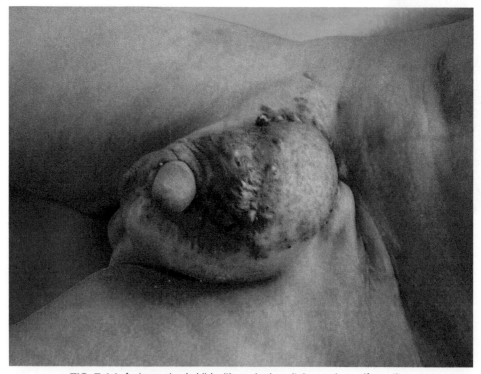

FIG. 7.14 A circumcised child with marked genital vascular malformation.

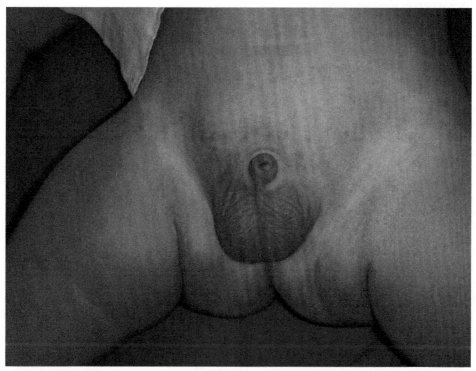

FIG. 7.15 A circumcised micropenis, which looks concealed after circumcision.

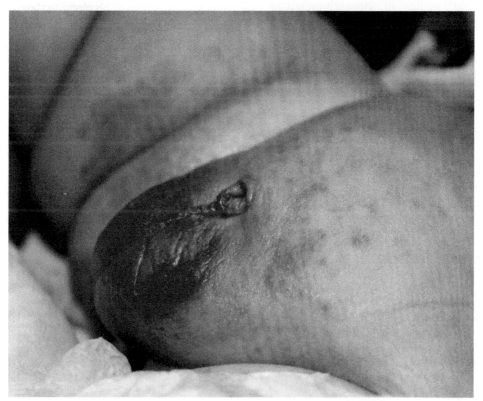

FIG. 7.16 A baby with an apparently concealed penis after circumcision due to the coexistence of an inguinal hernia.

- There is an obvious difference in the rate of MC complications between retrospective and prospective studies, with a low rate in the prospective studies because of improved procedures by practitioners or improved hygiene by patients as a result of participating in the study.
- The number of studies are small and the estimates of the frequency of complications will be correspondingly imprecise.
- Difference in the reported rates of complications is likely to be due to several factors directly associated with complications, such as age at circumcision, the training and expertise of the provider, the sterility of the conditions under which the procedure is performed and the indication (medical/cultural) for circumcision. In addition, there is variation due to methodological issues such as duration of follow-up, epidemiologic study design and definition of complications.
- Literature search found many case reports and case series of circumcision-related complications, but relatively few studies reported the proportion of circumcised males with a complication. For an accurate estimate of risks, active follow-up of circumcised boys is needed.
- Hospital-based studies of circumcision-related complications are usually retrospective and record based.

CLASSIFICATION OF MALE CIRCUMCISION COMPLICATIONS

There are different ways to classify post-MC complications: based on the severity, major and minor; based on the timing of detection of such complications, early and late (late complications are defined as those that occurred between 30 days and 5 years after circumcision); based on the extension in the human body, systemic and local; and based on the prevalence, common and rare.

It is difficult to report or to discuss one complication separately from others because many complications may be detected early after the procedure but have a late impact, such as an early local infection that may heal by fibrosis and result in penile curvature. Bleeding may be considered as a local complication, but if it is severe, it may end in a haemorrhagic shock. Meatal stenosis may also be considered as a rare complication in European countries, but it is so common in the developing communities with a high rate of neonatal MC.

Cases with abnormally nonaesthetic scar after MC are very difficult to be categorized, as overlapping of different forms and pathologic conditions is the rule. The surgeon may diagnose a case as incomplete circumcision but another one could call it as a CP or a case of cicatricial phimosis, so we opted herein to classify these complications under the heading 'nonaesthetic circumcision scar'.

A new classification of complications, initiated in 1992, is based on the type of therapy needed to correct the complication. The principle of this classification was to be simple, reproducible, flexible and applicable, irrespective of the cultural background; it is applied in grades from I to V according to their need for treatment.[21]

MC complications could be classified by using the Clavien-Dindo classification for surgical complications, in which the classes IIIa and IIIb refer to those complications with a need for surgical re-intervention and class IV for life-threatening complications. Another study proposed a classification of circumcision complications by separating them into five different grades: grade I, skin problems; grade II, isolated urethral lesion; grade III, amputation of the glans; grade IV, lesion of the corpus cavernosum; and grade V, total loss of the phallus.[22]

REFERENCES

1. Earp BD, Allareddy V, Rotta AT. Factors associated with early deaths following neonatal male circumcision in the United States, 2001 to 2010. *Clin Pediatr.* 2018;57(13). https://doi.org/10.1177/0009922818790060.
2. Okeke LI, Asinobi AA, Ikuerowo OS. Epidemiology of complications of male circumcision in Ibadan, Nigeria. *BMC Urol.* 2006;6:21.
3. Dave, et al. Guideline, foreskin care and neonatal circumcision in Canadian infants. *Can Urol Assoc J.* December 2017;1. https://doi.org/10.5489/cuaj.5033.
4. Perera CL, Bridgewater FH, Thavaneswaran P, et al. Safety and efficacy of nontherapeutic male circumcision: a systematic review. *Ann Fam Med.* 2010;8(1):64–72.
5. Weiss HA, Larke N, Halperin D, Schenker I. Complications of circumcision in male neonates, infants and children: a systematic review. *BMC Urol.* 2010;10:2. https://doi.org/10.1186/1471-2490-10-2. PMC 2835667.
6. Pieretti R, Goldstein A, Pieretti-Vanmarcke R. Late complications of newborn circumcision: a common and avoidable problem. *Pediatr Surg Int.* 2010;26:515–518.
7. El Bcheraoui C, Zhang X, Cooper CS, Rose CE, Kilmarx PH, Chen RT. Rates of adverse events associated with male circumcision in U.S. medical settings, 2001 to 2010. *JAMA Pediatr.* 2014;168:625–634. https://doi.org/10.1001/jamapediatrics.2013.5414. PMID: 24820907.
8. Horowitz M, Gershbein AB. Gomco circumcision: when is it safe? *J Pediatr Surg.* 2001;36(7):1047–1049.

9. Subramaniam R, Jacobsen AS. Sutureless circumcision: a prospective randomised controlled study. *Pediatr Surg Int.* 2004;20(10):783−785.

10. Mousavi SA, Salehifar E. Circumcision complications associated with the Plastibell device and conventional dissection surgery: a trial of 586 infants of ages up to 12 months. *Adv Urol.* 2008:606123.

11. Rodriguez V, Titapiwatanakun R, Moir C, et al. To circumcise or not to circumcise? Circumcision in patients with bleeding disorders. *Haemophilia.* 2009;16:272−276.

12. Storm DW, et al. The relationship between obesity and complications after neonatal circumcision. *J Urol.* 2011;186(Issue 4):1638−1641.

13. Akyol I, Soydan H, Kocoglu H, Ates F, Karademir K, Baykal K. A novel tool to predict the cosmetic outcome after circumcision: penile visibility index. *Int J Clin Med.* 2014;5:605−610.

14. Mayer E, Caruso DJ, Ankem M, Fisher MC, et al. Anatomic variants associated with newborn circumcision complications. *Can J Urol.* 2003;10(5):2013−2016.

15. Atikeler MK, Gecit I, Yuzgec V, Yalcin O. Complications of circumcision performed within and outside the hospital. *Int Urol Nephrol.* 2005;37(1):97−99.

16. Yegane RA, Kheirollahi AR, Salehi NA, Bashashati M, Khoshdel JA, Ahmadi M. Late complications of circumcision in Iran. *Pediatr Surg Int.* 2006;22(5):442−445.

17. Rehman J, Ghani M, Shehzad K, Sheikh I. Circumcision — a comparative study. *Pak Armed Forces Med J.* 2007;(4).

18. Palit V, Menebhi DK, Taylor I, Young M, Elmasry Y, Shah T. A unique service in UK delivering Plastibell (R) circumcision: review of 9-year results. *Pediatr Surg Int.* 2007;23(1):45−48.

19. Ozdemir E. Significantly increased complication risks with mass circumcisions. *Br J Urol.* 1997;80(1):136−139.

20. Thornton J. A randomized trial of Mogen clamp versus Plastibell for neonatal male circumcision in Botswana. *J Acquir Immune Defic Syndr.* 2013;64(2):e12−e13.

21. Dindo D, Demartines N, Clavien PA. Classification of surgical complications: a new proposal with evaluation in a cohort of 6336 patients and results of a survey. *Ann Surg.* August 2004;240(2):205−213 [PubMed].

22. Seleim HM, Elbarbary MM. Major penile injuries as a result of cautery during newborn circumcision. *J Pediatr Surg.* 2016;51(9):1532−1537 [PubMed].

CHAPTER 8

Bleeding Complications

MOHAMED A BAKY FAHMY, MD, FRCS

ABSTRACT

Bleeding is the most common complication of circumcision, and it is usually an immediate or early complication, with an incidence of 1% in a large retrospective review. There is variable incidence of post-circumcision bleeding reported in different studies, ranging between 4% and 35%. Roughly, excessive bleeding occurs in 1 in 1000 cases and it is usually treated with pressure or locally acting agents, but 1 in 4000 cases may require a ligature and 1 in 20,000 may need a blood transfusion, mostly because the child has a previously unrecognized bleeding disorder.

Bleeding could be major and leads to haemorrhagic shock or even death in rural areas, especially if the procedure is performed by nonmedical personnel, or if the baby had a bleeding tendency and his coagulation profile was not investigated before surgery. In patients with haemophilia who must undergo circumcision, preoperative and perioperative factor replacement is a definite requirement. Fibrin glue has been shown to decrease the amount of recombinant factor replacement needed (and also the cost of treatment) without significantly altering bleeding complications. Capillary, venous or, at times, arteriolar bleeding may occur; capillary bleeding usually settles with a firm dressing but the other two types may lead to exsanguination if not treated promptly.

KEYWORDS

Bipolar coagulation; Blood supply of the prepuce; Penile arteries; Venous drainage of the penis.

Bleeding is the most common complication of circumcision, and it is usually an immediate or early complication, with an incidence of 1% in a large retrospective review. There is variable incidence of post-circumcision bleeding reported in different studies, ranging between 4% and 35%. Roughly, excessive bleeding occurs in 1 in 1000 cases and it is usually treated with pressure or locally acting agents, but 1 in 4000 cases may require a ligature

and 1 in 20,000 may need a blood transfusion, mostly because the child has a previously unrecognized bleeding disorder.[1]

Bleeding could be major and leads to haemorrhagic shock or even death in rural areas, especially if the procedure is performed by nonmedical personnel, or if the baby had a bleeding tendency and his coagulation profile was not investigated before surgery. In patients with haemophilia who must undergo circumcision, preoperative and perioperative factor replacement is a definite requirement. Fibrin glue has been shown to decrease the amount of recombinant factor replacement needed (and also the cost of treatment) without significantly altering bleeding complications.[2] Capillary, venous or, at times, arteriolar bleeding may occur; capillary bleeding usually settles with a firm dressing, but the other two types may lead to exsanguination if not treated promptly.

Any physician who intended to practice male circumcision (MC) should be aware of the anatomy of the penis, especially its blood supply. Penile vasculature is completely different from any that of other organs, as erection merely relies on the penile blood supply.

BLOOD SUPPLY OF THE PENIS
Arteries

There are three paired main arteries in the penis: cavernosal, dorsal and bulbourethral (Fig. 8.1). All three arise from a shared branch of the internal pudendal artery, which arises from the internal iliac artery. On each side, the first branching occurs at the bulb of the spongiosum external to the urogenital diaphragm, forming the bulbourethral artery, which lies at the 9- and 3-o'clock positions of the corpus spongiosum. All three arteries communicate distally near the glans to provide an extensive anastomotic network.

Penile skin derives its supply from a separate origin; branches of the external pudendal artery supply the dorsal and lateral aspects of the penis and branches of the internal pudendal artery supply the ventral penis and scrotum via the posterior scrotal artery. The subcutaneous connective tissue of the penis

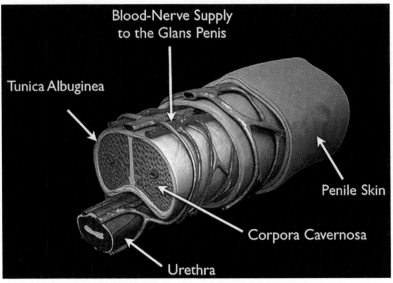

FIG. 8.1 Cross-sectional anatomy of penis.

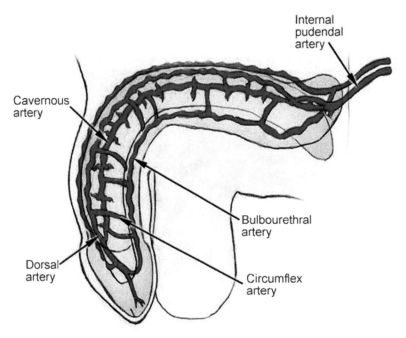

FIG. 8.2 Penile arteries.

and scrotum is called the dartos fascia, which continues into the perineum and fuses with the superficial perineal Colles fascia. The dartos fascia is loosely attached to the skin and the deep penile Buck fascia and contains the superficial arteries, veins and nerves of the penis (Fig. 8.2).

Venous Drainage

The penis is drained by 3 venous systems: the superficial, intermediate and deep veins (Fig. 8.3). Superficial veins are contained in the dartos fascia on the dorsolateral surface of the penis and coalesce at the base to form a single superficial dorsal vein, which usually drains

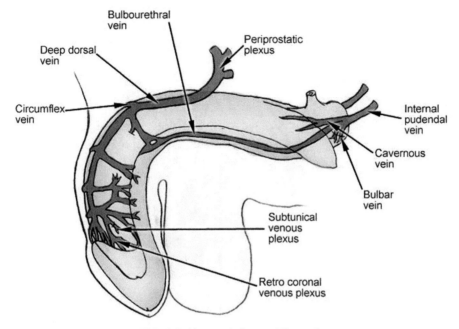

Bulbourethral
vein

Periprostatic
plexus

Deep dorsal
vein

Circumflex
vein

Internal
pudendal
vein

Cavernous
vein

Bulbar
vein

Subtunical
venous
plexus

Retro coronal
venous plexus

FIG. 8.3 Venous drainage of the penis.

into the great saphenous veins via the superficial external pudendal veins (Fig. 8.1).

The intermediate system contains the deep dorsal and the circumflex veins, lying within and beneath the Buck fascia. Emissary veins begin within the erectile tissue of the corpora cavernosa and drain into the circumflex or deep dorsal veins. The circumflex veins arise from the spongiosum, ventrum of the penis, and often the emissary veins drain into them.

The deep dorsal vein lies in the midline groove between the two corpora cavernosa and is formed from five to eight veins emerging from the glans penis, forming the retrocoronal plexus. It receives blood from the emissary and circumflex veins and passes underneath the symphysis pubis at the level of the suspensory ligament, leaving the shaft of the penis at the crus and draining into the prostatic plexus.

Deep venous drainage is via the crural and cavernosal veins. The crural veins arise in the midline, in the space between the crura. The cavernosal veins are consolidations of the emissary veins, which join to form a large venous channel that drains into the internal pudendal vein. Three or four small cavernosal veins course laterally between the corpus spongiosum and the

crus of the penis for 2–3 cm before draining into the internal pudendal veins.

Blood Supply to the Prepuce

Four arteries provide blood supply to the prepuce (Fig. 8.4). The inferior external pudendal artery gives off four branches as the superficial penile arteries (two enter the superficial fascia of the penis dorsolaterally and two enter it ventrolaterally). Beyond the preputial ring on the inner surface, the terminal branches become minute. These arteries are reflected towards the coronal sulcus where they anastomose with collaterals of the dorsal arteries. The blood supply to the frenulum arises from the dorsal arteries, which, at this point, have become dorsolateral.

At the level of the prepuce, certain branches are reflected to the anterior extremity towards the balanopreputial groove where they anastomose with the collaterals of the dorsal arteries. This is virtually the only point of anastomosis between the superficial and deep blood supply.

Venous drainage of the prepuce is less well organized (Fig. 8.4B). Multiple small veins in the prepuce without a particular orientation join the superficial dorsal veins and drain into the saphenous vein.

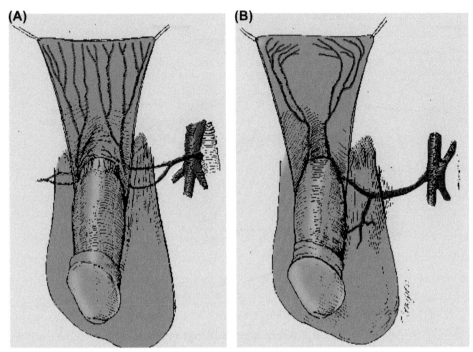

FIG. 8.4 (A) Arterial blood supply to the prepuce. (B) Venous drainage of the prepuce.

Magnitude of the Bleeding Complication

Bleeding after MC may be trivial and controllable in most cases, but in a few cases, especially in rural areas without medical facilities, it may end with a haemorrhagic shock and eventually death, if not promptly managed. Also, enthusiastic nonprofessional trials to stop post-MC bleeding are the cause of many subsequent lethal complications, such as glandular injury, urethral fistula and even entire penile gangrene. Rough manipulation and handling of the penile tissues may predispose to post-circumcision infection and granuloma formation, which may be again superimposed by a late bleeding.

CLASSIFICATION OF POST-MALE CIRCUMCISION BLEEDING

Preoperative Bleeding

Bleeding is rarely reported at the anaesthetic site during dorsal nerve block or ring block, and it is manifested as a bruise or haematoma at the injection site, which usually will subside by gentle compression or fomentation (Fig. 8.5). Shaft haematoma due to either puncture of superficial dorsal vein at the time of injecting local anaesthetic or retraction of vein while performing a dorsal slit at the time of insertion of Plastibell may persist for a couple of days, and usually annoys the parents.

More investigation to rule out bleeding tendency and frequent compression is mandatory (Fig. 8.6).

A rough preputial retraction, especially in neonates with the common physiologic phimosis, by an inexperienced circumcisor usually results in frenular bleeding, which could be stopped by genital compression. Any attempt to use cautery in this area, especially a unipolar one, may result in urethral fistula (Fig. 8.7) (this will be discussed in Chapter 12, Figs 12.12 and 12.13).

Intraoperative Bleeding

During MC procedure, bleeding is commonly trivial and occurs at the dorsal or frenular vessels. Gentle compression, fine ligature or use of bipolar diathermy could control bleeding in most cases. Bleeding from the edges of both outer and inner preputial layers is usually controlled by interrupted absorbable stitching, and compression bandage applied by some physicians to control such bleeding may result in haematoma formation. Frenular bleeding occurs if Plastibell rubs against the fastidious frenular area, while the baby excessively moves his legs. Wound oozing recognized and controlled at the hospital or at the scene of circumcision is not considered as a complication.

Bleeding during MC is usually common after dissection in the improper plane, especially at the ventral

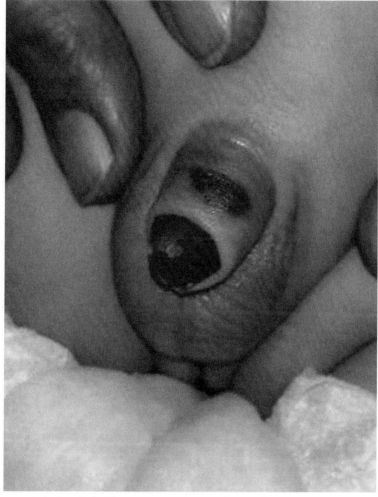

FIG. 8.5 Dorsal haematoma at the site of local anaesthetic injection.

surface of the glans or coronal sulcus, and several trials to stop bleeding by using heavy instrument or rough tissue handling will end in more complications, such as tissue necrosis, glandular loss and urethral injury (Fig. 8.8).

Postoperative Bleeding

Bleeding either immediately after the procedure or later on is commonly seen after slipping of bandage or ligatures, as well as in patients with unrecognized bleeding tendency. Late bleeding may follow fall of a crust or scab covering a significant vessel, where the bleeding may occur along the skin edges between sutures, or from a discrete blood vessel, most commonly at the frenulum (Fig. 8.9).

Meticulous attention to haemostasis during an open procedure and adequate time for skin edge compression during newborn circumcisions may prevent haemorrhage in the majority of cases. Post-circumcision bleeding can be controlled by applying direct pressure or careful application of compressive bandage. Rarely, wound exploration and suturing is necessary in some cases. Hospital admission, assessment of the haemodynamic status, proper investigation + blood transfusion and insertion of a urethral catheter to avoid urine retention are our policies to deal with all cases of post-MC bleeding, especially if MC was performed by nonmedical personnel outside hospitals or during mass circumcision (Fig. 8.10). Wound exploration under general anaesthesia and securing haemostasis with fine stitches with a low current bipolar diathermy is indicated in all cases with significant bleeding or with a large haematoma.

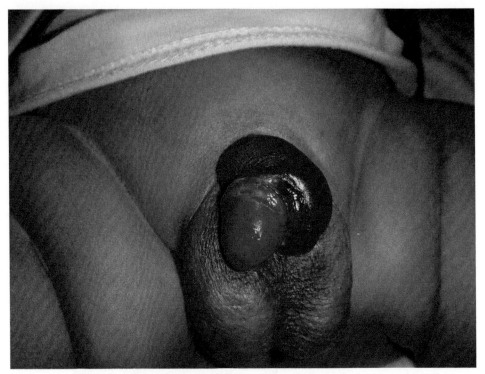

FIG. 8.6 Resistant significant shaft haematoma.

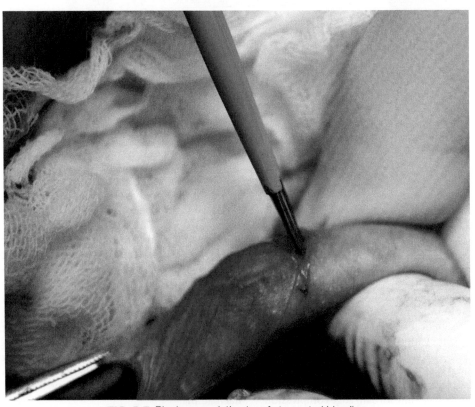

FIG. 8.7 Bipolar coagulation is safe to control bleeding.

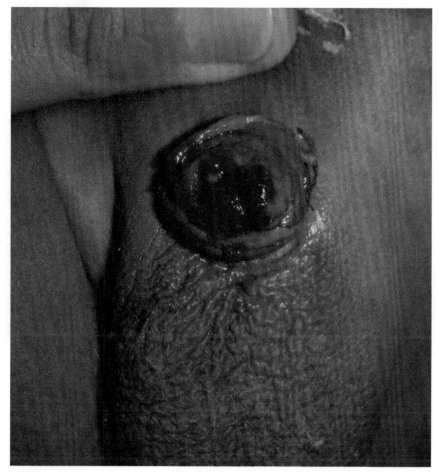

FIG. 8.8 Glans penis injury resulting in considerable bleeding, and usually, it leads to glandular tissue loss or late disfigurement.

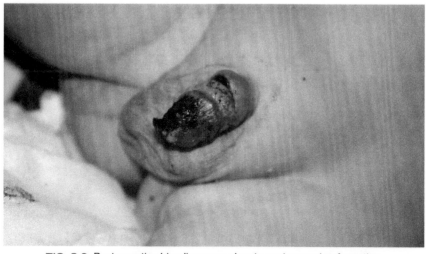

FIG. 8.9 Postoperative bleeding secondary to cautery eschar formation.

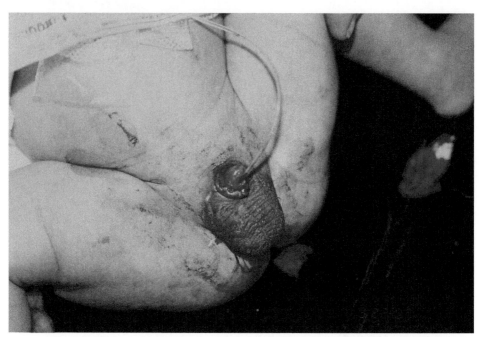

FIG. 8.10 Major bleeding necessitates hospital admission and urinary catheter insertion.

REFERENCES

1. Avanoglu A, elik AC, Ulman I, et al. Safer circumcision in patients with haemophilia: the use of fibrin glue for local haemostasis. *BJU Int.* 1999;83(1):91–94.

2. Rodriguez RT, Moir C, Schmidt KA, Pruthi RK. To circumcise or not to circumcise? Circumcision in patients with bleeding disorders. *Haemophilia.* 2010;16(2):272–276.

CHAPTER 9

Infectious Complications of Circumcision

MOHAMED A BAKY FAHMY, MD, FRCS

ABSTRACT

Although uncommon, local, systemic and toxin-related infectious complications of circumcision represent a significant clinical problem. In general, untrained providers create more infectious and noninfectious complications when performing male circumcision than well-trained providers, regardless of whether they are physicians, nurses or traditional religious providers. Local infections include staphylococcal and streptococcal infections, cellulitis, impetigo, pyoderma, necrotizing fasciitis, scalded skin syndrome (staphylococcal), Fournier gangrene, glanular necrosis, scrotal abscess and even peritonitis. Systemic infectious complications include bacteraemia, meningitis, pneumonia or septicaemia, and rare incidence of tuberculosis and diphtheria had been reported, but the frequency of reporting such cases had declined.

KEYWORDS

Balanitis; Candida balanitis; Fournier gangrene; Meatal stenosis; Meatal ulcers; Meatitis; Penile granuloma; Smegma granuloma; Suture granulomas.

The infectious complications of circumcision include
- Post-circumcision penile granuloma,
- Post-male circumcision (MC) balanitis,
- Post-MC meatitis,
- Meatal ulcers,
- Meatal stenosis,
- Fournier gangrene.

Although uncommon, local, systemic and toxin-related infectious complications of circumcision represent a significant clinical problem. In general, untrained providers create more infectious and noninfectious complications when performing MC than well-trained providers, regardless of whether they are physicians, nurses or traditional religious providers. Local infections include staphylococcal and streptococcal infections, cellulitis, impetigo, pyoderma, necrotizing fasciitis, scalded skin syndrome (staphylococcal), Fournier gangrene, glanular necrosis, scrotal abscess and even peritonitis. Systemic infectious complications include bacteraemia, meningitis, pneumonia or septicaemia, and rare incidence of tuberculosis and diphtheria had been reported, but the frequency of reporting such cases had declined.[1]

INCIDENCE

Owing to the superb dual blood supply of the penis, wound infection occurs infrequently. Gee and Ansell[2] studied a series of 5521 circumcisions in developed countries comparing the Plastibell technique with the Gomco clamp and reported only 23 (0.4%) cases of infectious complications, and of those cases, the Plastibell group had significantly more infections. In another study, however, the Plastibell method had less chances of infection (4%) as compared with the open method (10%).[3] There is no precise estimation of the actual rate of post-MC infection in many developing countries, and a few studies published from some centers usually report based on short-term follow-up.

PATHOLOGY

Several factors may contribute to the different presentations of post-circumcision infection, especially in developing countries where there are no guidelines for performing the procedure and aseptic conditions are not usually available or not followed:
- The raw glandular surface after rough forcible separation of the prepuce from the glans in neonates may pave the way for a pathogenic organism to induce local or systemic infection (Fig. 9.1).
- Skin loss leaving a bared penile shaft due to extensive removal of the penile skin (degloving injury) in neonates, especially in buried, concealed and webbed penises, usually results in different grades of post-MC infection (Fig. 9.2).

Complications in Male Circumcision. https://doi.org/10.1016/B978-0-323-68127-8.00009-0

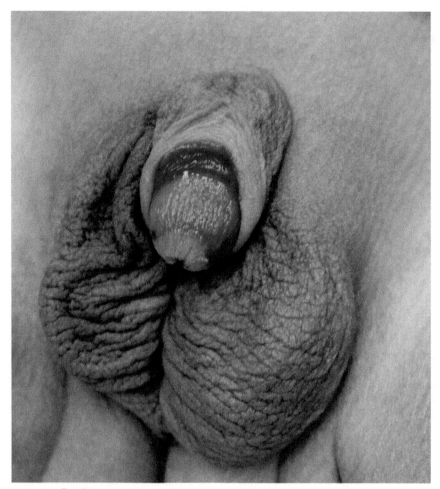

FIG. 9.1 Forcible preputial retraction in a neonate usually results in raw glandular surface.

- Extensive improper use of thermal or unipolar cautery may cause tissue devastation, paving the way for secondary infection (Fig. 9.3).

- Injurious tissue necrosis secondary to ischaemia in a small neonate or in those who are immunocompromised may result in a condition similar to Fournier gangrene, which is very difficult to manage and may eventually leads to penile loss (Fig. 9.4).

- Severe infections following Plastibell circumcision, including necrotizing fasciitis,[3] have also been reported, probably due to more tight tie, retained ring or improper ring size (Fig. 9.5).

- Heavy stitches and post-circumcision bleeding complicated with a haematoma and tissue ischaemia commonly predispose to a pyogenic penile infection (Fig. 9.6).

- Causative organisms are usually the skin flora, but because of the uniquely dirty environment of the diaper, colonic flora has also been reported. *Pseudomonas aeruginosa* infection is the most serious one, which results in severe tissue necrosis (Fig. 9.7).

- Fungal or candida infection does not rarely complicate neonatal MC. It may be seen especially in a debilitated child with bad napkin hygiene, or in those with diabetes (Fig. 9.8).

- Lethal tetanus infection after neonatal circumcision was reported in some areas.[4]

Several authors described the presenting signs and symptoms as erythema, induration, pain out of proportion to physical findings, coupled with tachycardia, leucocytosis or bandemia. As in adults, infection is usually polymicrobial, but in severe cases, pus or a pyogenic

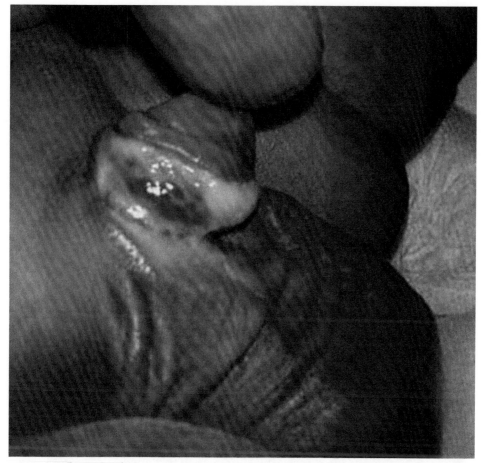

FIG. 9.2 Pyogenic infection, secondary to extensive skin removal from the lateral penile surface.

membrane may be detectable a few days after circumcision (Figs. 9.2 and 9.6).

Infection is usually mild and manifested by local inflammatory changes, which typically resolve with local topical triple antibiotic ointment. However, ulceration, suppuration and systemic infection (e.g. sepsis and meningitis) can occur and should be suspected in cases with systemic symptoms, such as fever, irritability, lethargy or poor feeding.[5]

Although urinary tract infection (UTI) can occur in circumcised male infants, the frequency of UTI is significantly lower in circumcised infants than in uncircumcised infants (0.02% vs. 0.19%).[6] So UTI is not a complication of circumcision, but rather, a reduced risk of UTI is a benefit of this procedure. In Jewish ritual circumcision, and in other African countries, tightly wrapped gauze is used to stop minor bleeding (as compared with the use of local pressure in hospitals), and it is thought that this can cause urinary retention

and hence UTI. Severe and extensive post-MC infection may result in urinary retention due to glandular oedema and meatal obstruction, such cases may need catheterization, with the possibility of infection spreading (Fig. 9.9).

Persistent ulceration of the glans penis may follow inadequate treatment of post-circumcision infection (Fig. 9.10), and a late sequelae of bending and penile curvature could follow some cases of severe penile infection.

Fournier gangrene will be discussed with ischaemic vascular complications (see Chapter 12).

PREVENTION

Most infections can be prevented by proper patient preparation, glove wearing and good local wound care including cleaning the penis and post-MC application of antibiotic ointment with frequent diaper changes.

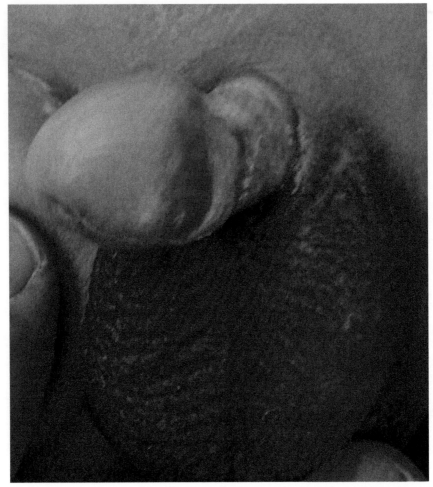

FIG. 9.3 Extensive skin loss from the penile shaft after improper use of diathermy, followed by infection.

Also post-circumcision care is mandatory not only by the mothers to look after the wound by cleaning and avoiding soiling with stool but also by physicians to follow-up the baby, to pick up any early complications and to manage them accordingly.

TREATMENT

Local infections are easily treated with local antibiotics, whereas systemic infections require intravenous or intramuscular injectable antibiotics. Empirical broad-spectrum antibiotics to treat gram-negative, gram-positive and anaerobic organisms are essential in cases suspected to have an extensive local or systemic infection. A suggested regimen is an aminoglycoside, nafcillin, or vancomycin and clindamycin. Prompt surgical evaluation and early aggressive debridement of necrotic tissue are required, and for complicated cases, remedy with appropriate penile reconstruction could be planned later. Hyperbaric oxygen may be indicated in some cases, and it will be discussed in Chapter 13.

POST-CIRCUMCISION PENILE GRANULOMA

Some complications of circumcision cannot be avoided, even when the procedure is carried out by trained surgeons. Although infection is not uncommon after circumcision, the implantation of a foreign body, e.g. talcum powder, excess suture material or smegma particles, during circumcision may induce an abnormal tissue response later on, with the development of granulation tissue concomitant to infectious complications.

The development of post-circumcision penile granuloma was described well in a large series by

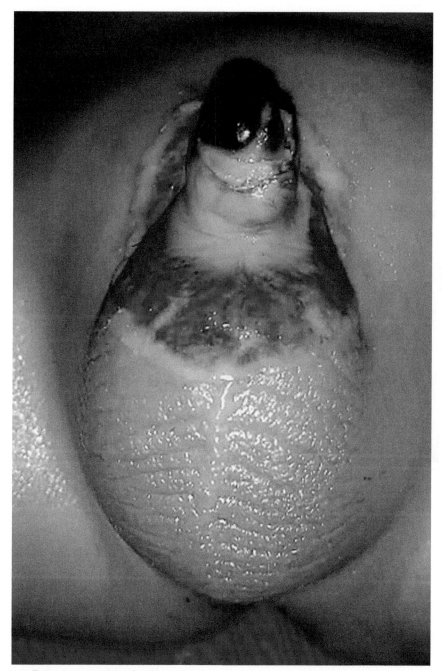

FIG. 9.4 Extensive necrotizing fasciitis and ischaemia in a neonate, which ended in Fournier gangrene.

Atikeler et al.,[7] in which 26 cases of different granulomas (5%) were found in 523 circumcised boys, with a mean time to develop granuloma of 3.2 months after MC. The cause of post-circumcision granuloma has been postulated to be due to a foreign body (e.g. talcum powder, excess suture material or smegma particles), which may be introduced during circumcision between preputial layers, resulting in a tissue response manifested as a granuloma of different sizes and types.

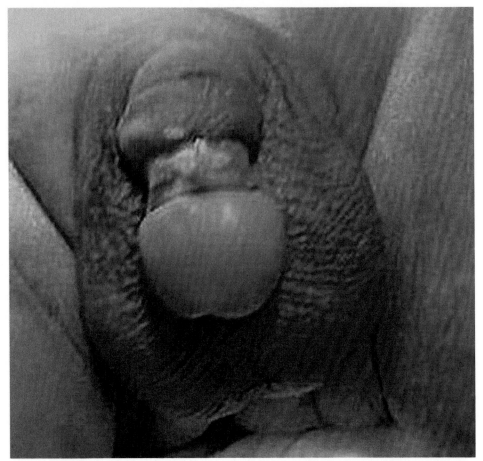

FIG. 9.5 Subcoronal infection and necrosis, secondary to prolonged retention of the Plastibell ring.

POST-MC GRANULOMA COULD BE MANIFESTED AS IN THE FOLLOWING

- Pyogenic granuloma: Localized chronic infection may result in pyogenic granuloma, which may be presented as a small growth with a characteristic granular surface, bleeds on touch and can be managed with local dressing (Fig. 9.11), but a large granuloma is rarely diagnosed after MC and meticulous surgical excision is necessary in such cases. (Fig. 9.12).
- Suture granulomas: This is a reaction to the stitches that did not dissolve as intended. It appears as bumps of different sizes under the skin around the wound as the skin creates a tiny wall of scar tissue around the suture to separate it from the body. Suture granuloma could be recognized early after circumcision or later, after weeks or even months (Fig. 9.13).

Microscopically, foreign body granuloma to suture material (nylon, silk and sometimes dyed polyglycolic) contains multinucleated giant cells, with haphazardly arranged nuclei. These giant cells are fused macrophages. The foreign body is birefringent and may sometimes be visible by polarized light in the middle of the granuloma or inside the giant cells.

- Smegma granuloma: Small particles of smegma may persist between the edges of a circumcision wound. If the particles are not removed before cutting the prepuce, they may form a small granuloma at the circumcised penile skin edges (Fig. 9.13), but under unknown circumstances, smegma may form a well-formed cyst or cysts of larger sizes (Chapter 10, Figs 31–34).

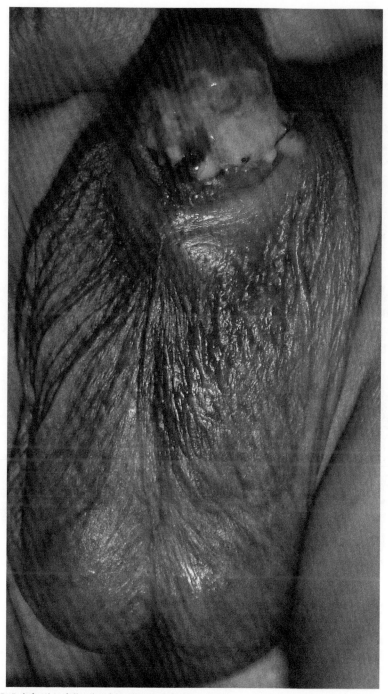

FIG. 9.6 Infection following bleeding and heavy stitching, with associated scrotal haematoma.

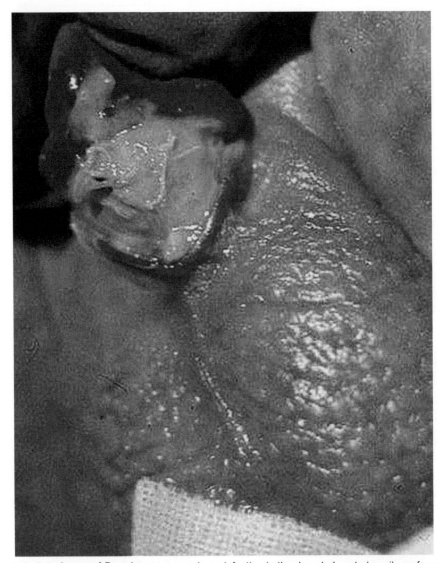

FIG. 9.7 A case of *Pseudomonas aeruginosa* infection in the denuded ventral penile surface.

CLINICAL MANIFESTATION

The granuloma, if not treated early, it may become larger and will be troublesome to both the baby and his mother, discharging mucous with irritation and pain and it may bleed with napkin contact (Fig. 9.14).

TREATMENT

It is usually conservative, as many of these lesions may resolve spontaneously. Frequent washing and dressing with polyurethane (Lyofoam), topical doxycycline and topical clobetasol propionate cream 0.05% may be indicated for resistant cases.

Silver nitrate: Large granulomas not responding to conservative measures may need silver nitrate cauterization, which acts as an antiseptic, an astringent and a caustic agent. Conventional management was to dry the granuloma and carefully cauterize it with a 75% silver nitrate stick, but great caution should be paid to avoid spillage to the normal surrounding tissues (Fig. 9.15A and B).

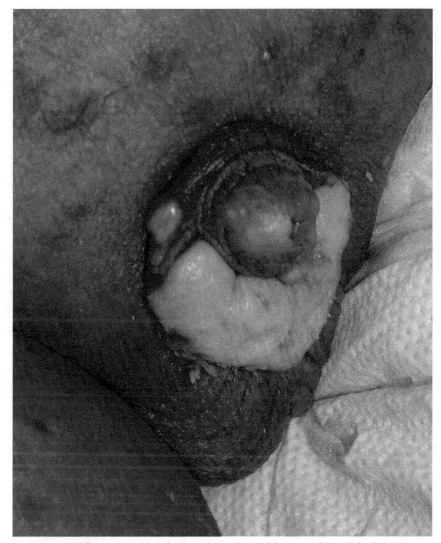

FIG. 9.8 Severe candida infection of the circumcision wound in a diabetic baby.

Surgical excision could be the mainstay of treatment for large or non-resolving granuloma after chemical cauterization, with fine suturing of skin edges to avoid recurrence, and great caution should be exerted to avoid injury of the underlying tissue, especially the urethra.

Wide area of skin loss after MC may also heal with a granulation tissue and may subsequently result in different forms of penile curvature or bending after healing with fibrosis (Fig. 9.16).

POST-MALE CIRCUMCISION BALANITIS

Balanitis is defined as inflammation of the glans penis, which often involves the prepuce; in such cases, it is called balanoposthitis and is not rare in uncircumcised men. Balanitis is a common condition affecting 11% of men attending the genitourinary clinic, and it could be a recurrent or persistent condition.[8]

Clinically balanitis presents with mild burning, pruritus, itching, swelling, erythematous patches and plaques or bullae involving the glans penis, as well as satellite eroded pustules and moist curd-like accumulations may be seen in a few cases. Balanitis has worse clinical presentation in diabetic and immunocompromised patients, with a fulminating oedema or ulcers in severe cases.

There is a wide variety of causes and predisposing factors that lead to the development of balanitis, such

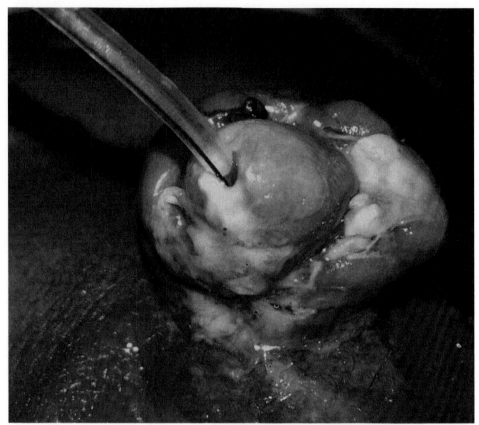

FIG. 9.9 Severe post-male circumcision infection results in urinary retention and necessitates catheterization.

as poorer hygiene and aeration of the genital area or smegma irritation. People with underlying medical conditions, such as diabetics and immunocompromised patients, may be more vulnerable to different forms and extension of balanitis. Also excessive glandular destruction by the thermal effect of diathermy and impertinent tissue handling may pave the way for secondary infection and balanitis after MC (Fig. 9.17).

Balanitis has been reported as a source of fever and bacteraemia in neutropenic men, and candida balanitis may be especially severe in patients with diabetes mellitus. While inflammation of the penis may occur more frequently in circumcised boys, balanoposthitis in the normal penis may be more painful because the nerve endings in the prepuce are sensitive to fine touch.

Most paediatricians often mislabel balanitis as 'candida diaper rash or contact dermatitis'. When the circumcision scar and glans are the focus of infection, different grades of balanitis may complicate the procedure. In a large retrospective study, the incidence of balanitis in circumcised and uncircumcised boys did not

differ significantly. But in another study, balanitis or irritation was documented in 4% of uncircumcised boys up to age 12 years, compared with 10.4% in circumcised boys of the same age. It appears that circumcised boys <10 years old are more likely to develop balanitis than normal boys.[9]

I think post-neonatal MC balanitis is an underestimated complication, especially in developing countries, as most of the babies are not followed up properly by the physicians after the procedure, and if they are followed up, this is usually done once in the first week. It is proposed that the naked glans is liable to different forms of infections after removal of the prepuce (Fig. 9.1), especially if the napkins are not changed frequently and proper care for the circumcision wound is not followed by the mothers, and also concomitant gastroenteritis and diarrhoea, which are still not uncommon in developing countries, may aggravate the condition and predispose to different forms of balanitis that may progress to urinary meatus and result in meatitis, UTI, meatal ulcers or stenosis.

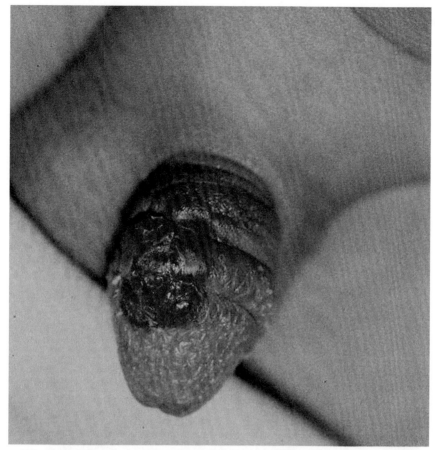

FIG. 9.10 Post-circumcision infectious large ulcer over the glans and coronal sulcus.

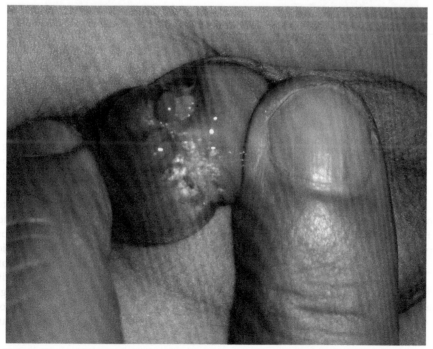

FIG. 9.11 A small granuloma in coronal sulcus developed 2 weeks after male circumcision.

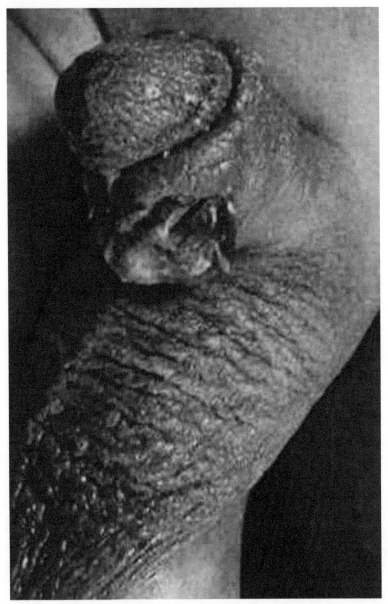

FIG. 9.12 A large granuloma in the ventral penile surface.

Post-MC balanitis could be bacterial or fungal, but rarely a specific form of balanitis xerotica obliterans (BXO) may supervene MC, especially at older ages.

BACTERIAL OR PYOGENIC BALANITIS

Bacterial or pyogenic balanitis is not rare after MC. The common organism involved is *Streptococcus* and less common ones are *Haemophilus parainfluenzae, Klebsiella, Staphylococcus epidermidis, Enterococcus, Proteus, Morganella* and *Escherichia coli*, which may be detected in cases of combined infection (Fig. 9.9).

Local measures with frequent dressing may be enough to cure most cases, but a few cases may need systemic antibiotics.

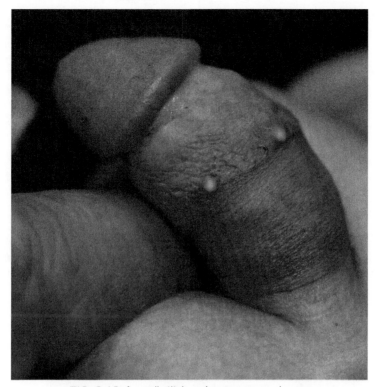

FIG. 9.13 A small stitch and smegma granulomas.

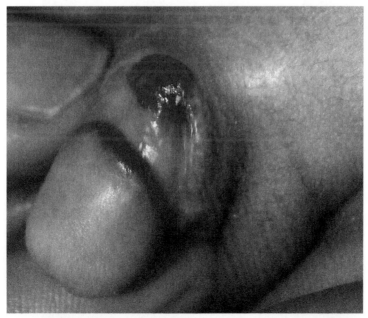

FIG. 9.14 Infected granuloma at the dorsum of circumcision scar.

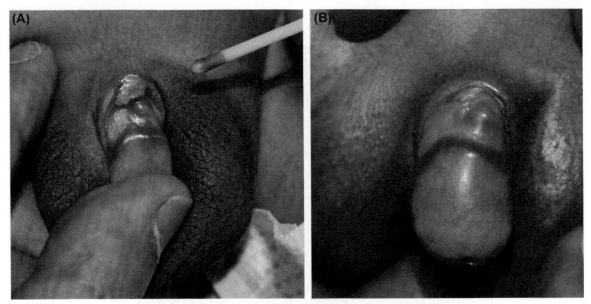

FIG. 9.15 (A, B) The same case in Fig. 9.14 managed by silver nitrate stick cauterization with complete resolution.

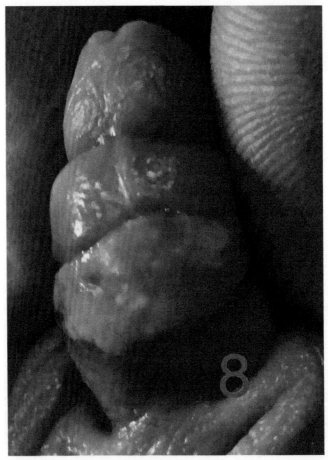

FIG. 9.16 Wide area of subcoronal granulation after excessive penile skin loss, which may heal with fibrosis and subsequent bending.

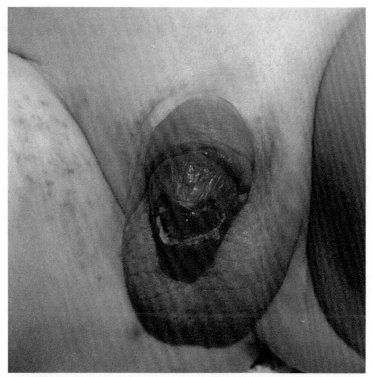

FIG. 9.17 Deep glandular ulcer after falling down of the post-male circumcision injury crust, which may predispose to secondary balanitis.

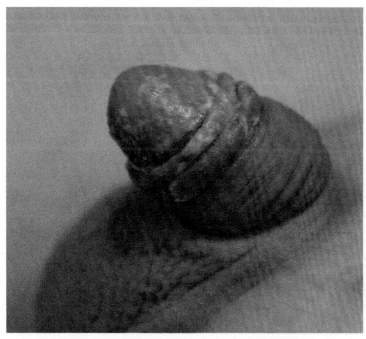

FIG. 9.18 Post-male circumcision fungal balanitis.

FUNGAL OR CANDIDA BALANITIS

Candida albicans is the most frequent fungi isolated from the penis. Fungi are a normal flora but their overgrowth can occur in certain conditions, especially in diabetic patients with phimosis. Candida colonization was seen in 16% of men visiting a sexually transmitted infection clinic in Coventry, United Kingdom.[9] Symptomatic infection due to *C. albicans* is more common in uncircumcised males. Bacterial superinfection with streptococci or staphylococci increases pain.

I believe that fungal and candida balanitis are more common than the bacterial one, due to the soiling of the circumcision wound with stool or the surrounding environment. In children, most cases were aged 2−5 years, had a red rash and sometimes had white, shiny patches on the glans penis. The skin on the penis

may be moist and a thick white substance may be detected (Fig. 9.18). At older age, infection may occur without sexual contact, usually in the presence of diabetes.

Diagnosis may be done based on clinical appearance alone, without microscopy or tissue culture, as the sensitivity of microscopy varies with the method of sampling, and an "adhesive tape" method has proven to be more accurate than swabbing.

TREATMENT OF BALANITIS

These cases usually respond well to topical antifungal medications, and systemic forms are rarely indicated. Topical antifungals, if applied consistently until symptoms disappear, may be effective in the treatment of

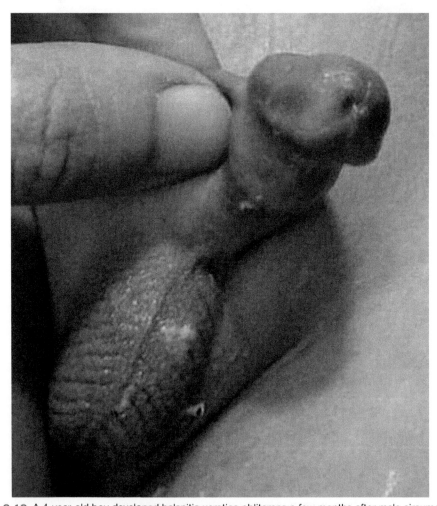

FIG. 9.19 A 4-year-old boy developed balanitis xerotica obliterans a few months after male circumcision.

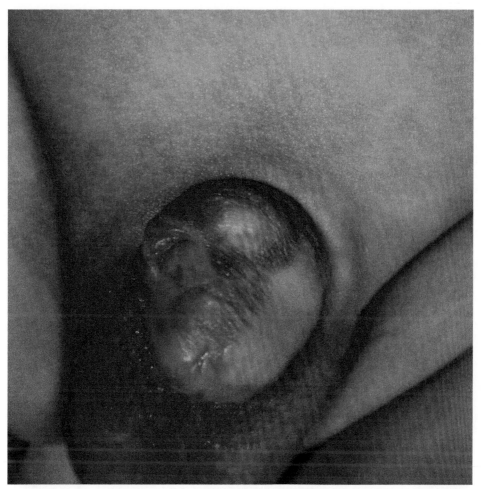

FIG. 9.20 A 3-year-old boy with extensive scaring and meatal affection due to balanitis xerotica obliterans after circumcision.

most cases. Recurrence is frequent, however, especially in patients with risk factors such as diabetes. Treatment of the partner is important to reduce the risk of relapse in sexually active adults.

POST-CIRCUMCISION BALANITIS XEROTICA OBLITERANS

It is generally rare in children younger than 5 years. It was described for the first time in 1928 by Stuhmer, and it is considered as the male genital variant of lichen sclerosus. The name was derived from the three components of the disease: balanitis, 'chronic inflammation of the glans penis', xerotic, 'abnormally dry appearance of the lesion'; and obliterans, 'the association of occasional endarteritis'.[10]

Most publications consider BXO as the disease of uncircumcised men and usually circumcision is highly indicated as a line of treatment for most cases, but this is not accurately true because many cases of BXO may be seen after MC, even a few cases were diagnosed with BXO after glans penis amputation.[11]

We diagnosed a few cases of different forms of BXO after MC. It is not known if this rare disease complicates MC or if it could exist, as a mild form, before the procedure and may only be manifested later on after circumcision. Such cases will present after a few months with glans discolouration, mainly in the form of white plaques, with red area in between but with no ulceration; itching and burning are common, and difficult micturition is the main complaint if the meatus and/or urethra is affected by the disease progression

(Fig. 9.19). Severe scaring and glandular distortion are very rare after MC (Fig. 9.20).

In one study, BXO was diagnosed in 9% of 100 consecutive circumcisions performed for religious reasons and in 19% of 232 circumcisions performed for disease of the prepuce and penis.[12]

The disease mainly affects the prepuce in uncircumcised men, and glandular involvement occurs in 49% of cases. Although the meatus is affected in a variable proportion, it causes severe tissue destruction and often causes meatal stenosis and urethral stricture.

The cause of BXO has not yet been determined; there is no identified viral or bacterial cause or familial predisposition. The association of BXO and penile cancer in children is also not established.[13]

Histologic examination of the excised tissue usually confirms the diagnosis, showing hyperkeratosis with follicular plugging, atrophy of the stratum spongiosum Malpighi with hydropic degeneration of basal cells, lymphoedema, hyalinosis, acanthosis and homogenization of collagen in the upper dermis and inflammatory infiltration in the mid-dermis.[13] On the basis of the evolution of the disease and the histopathologic features, the lesions were classified into early, established and advanced forms.

TREATMENT

Various treatments are described, but there is no consensus on which one is the best. Treatment options include medical and surgical management. The use of topical corticosteroids has had limited benefit in treating BXO, with scar formation. Children with meatal involvement should be observed frequently because of the risk of recurrent meatal stenosis. In boys presenting with milder forms of BXO, the application of a potent topical steroid (e.g. 0.05% mometasone furoate, 0.05% clobetasol propionate or 0.05% betamethasone

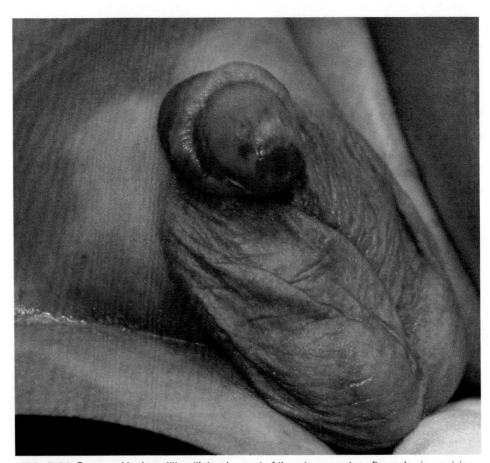

FIG. 9.21 Sever napkin dermatitis with involvement of the urinary meatus after male circumcision.

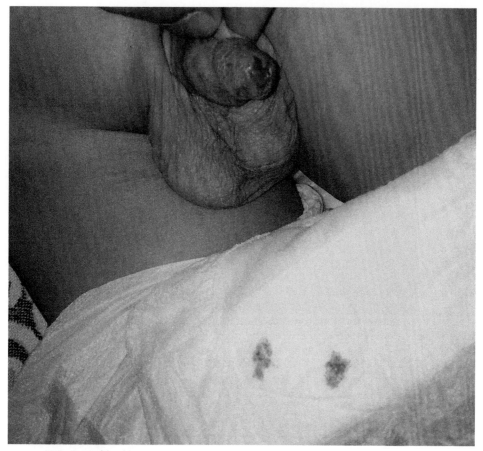

FIG. 9.22 Meatitis secondary to male circumcision presented with urethral bleeding.

cream) may ameliorate local symptoms and result in an improvement in the appearances of the glans. Meatoplasty is the most common urinary reconstructive surgery associated with BXO. Even though it is not frequently needed, it is described in up to 36% of patients from paediatric urology centers.[10]

POST-MALE CIRCUMCISION MEATITIS

There is an increasing attention paid to a peculiar lesion of the meatus urinarius, occurring only in circumcised male children and characterized by ulceration, crusting, narrowing of the urinary passage and nearly always accompanied by painful urination, often with distended bladder and occasionally with haemorrhages. It is usually a manifestation of post-MC meatitis.

It is difficult to distinguish the three pathologic entities affecting the meatus in circumcised boys: meatitis, meatal ulcer and meatal stricture. The pathologic condition may start as meatitis and develop into a meatal ulcer, which eventually results in meatal stricture. Cases detected early and treated promptly may be aborted early after meatitis without the sequence of stenosis.

Habitually; the exposed meatus is the only seat of a diaper lesion, rarely it is spared. As a rule, it is involved with the rest of the diaper region.[14]

Unless special care and proper hygiene are applied to the exposed urinary meatus after ritual MC, it will be vulnerable to ammoniacal dermatitis (meatitis), napkin dermatitis and other pathologic forms (Fig. 9.21).

Meatitis may be manifested by burning micturition, itching or urethral bleeding (Fig. 9.22).

In a few cases, meatal or glandular injuries and ischaemia, due to different causes, if not cared properly, may be complicated with pyogenic infection around the urinary meatus, which may be extended to the distal urethra. Such cases should be managed carefully with

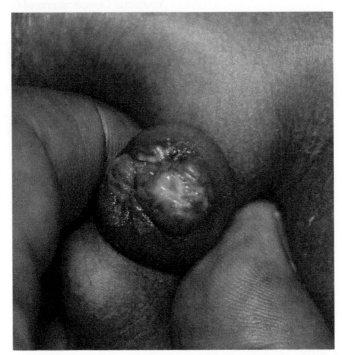

FIG. 9.23 A case of pyogenic meatitis complicating meatal and glandular injury, after guillotine male circumcision.

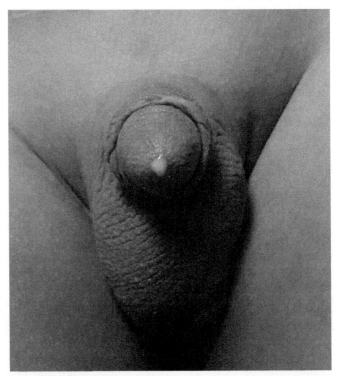

FIG. 9.24 A case of *Streptococcus pyogenes* meatitis detected 2 weeks after male circumcision with a frank pus discharge from the meatus.

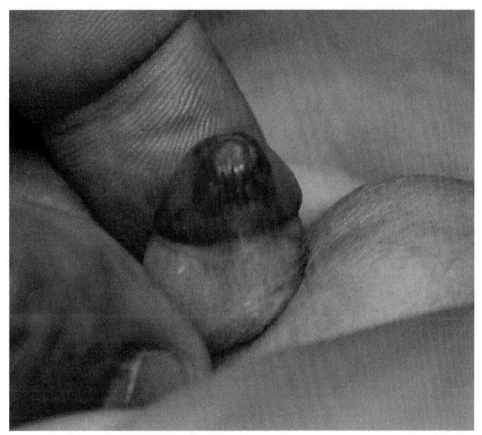

FIG. 9.25 Severe meatitis, which necessitated biopsy to rule out other specific pathologic conditions.

proper antibiotics and frequent dressing and special attention has to be paid during follow-up to avoid any supervening meatal stricture (Fig. 9.23).

Also many cases diagnosed as balanitis, if not treated properly, may end with a localized infection of the meatus. Appreciation of frank pus discharge from the meatus is not common among children, and in such cases, a specific organism, such as *Streptococcus pyogenes*, or other rare bacteria could be isolated (Fig. 9.24).

Swabs should be taken from any suspected case to determine the causative organisms, as many cases will respond well to local care with proper hygiene, but local and rarely systemic antibiotics may be indicated. Suspicious cases that do not respond to simple measures of treatment, or are extensive from the beginning, should undergo biopsy to rule out specific causes such as BXO, Zoon (plasma cell) balanitis or other dermatosis (Fig. 9.25).

MEATAL ULCERS

Superficial ulceration of the urethral meatus is a definite entity occurring in male infants and young boys after MC, and in spite of its frequent incidence, little was known about it. It occurs chiefly in circumcised children and may also be found in non-circumcised children if the prepuce leaves the tip of the glans free to irritation. This disease was first noted by J. von Bokay[15] in 1878 in 23 boys who were all Jewish and circumcised. He called the lesion 'urethritis orificii externi'. He believed that the condition was due to poor hygiene but expressed the opinion that it may also be due to certain irritating qualities of the urine.

Ulceration of the meatus in circumcised infants of the diaper age is common. It is practically restricted to artificially fed infants from 5 to 18 months of age, and it is caused by free ammonia on the night diaper. The narrowed meatus is clearly a result and not a cause of the ulceration. Studies have found meatal ulcerations in 8%–31% of circumcised boys.[16]

The ulcer always remains superficial and localized and never involves the deeper parts of the urethra. Urethral discharge rarely occurs and there is no fever. The inguinal lymph nodes are sometimes swollen and tender. Crusts may form rapidly on the surface of the ulcer and may partially or completely obstruct the meatus, leading to difficulty in voiding and is therefore usually followed by urinary retention (Fig. 9.26).

More commonly the lesion manifests itself as a rather superficial ulceration about the meatus, but at times, the ulcer becomes deep and extensive, measuring up to 2 mm in depth and more than 5 mm in width. Usually it is more or less covered by a crust that is very firmly attached over a considerable area. Surrounding the ulcer, there is often an area of inflammation that involves both the adjacent surface of the glans and extends into the urethral opening with consequent narrowing. In severe cases, there is commonly an association among erythema, vesication (minute blistering) and ulceration of the glans, scrotum and the rest of the diaper region wherever the diaper is in extensive contact with the skin (Fig. 9.27). A permanent narrowing of the meatus, analogous to a stricture, apparently rarely occurs even after repeated and prolonged ulceration.

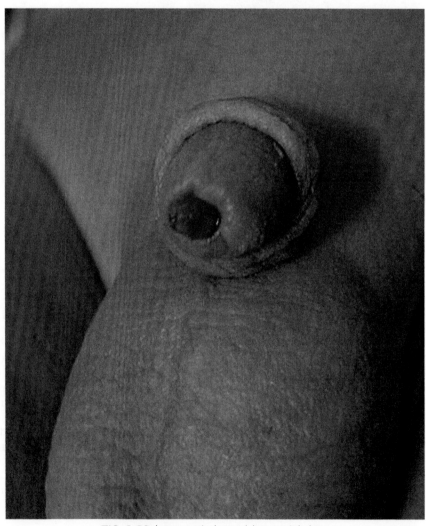

FIG. 9.26 Large post-circumcision meatal ulcer.

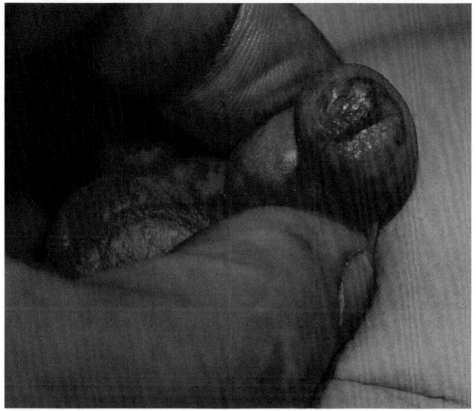

FIG. 9.27 Meatitis with erythema and vesication (minute blistering) around the meatus after male circumcision.

MEATAL STENOSIS

Most patients in whom the lesion is recognized are children. In practically all of whom it may be considered congenital, acquired cases are not common and are usually seen in circumcised boys. The normal urethral meatus is 10F before 4 years of age, 12F from 4 to 10 years of age and 14F after 10 years of age. Because of its high incidence, the risk of developing meatal stenosis needs to be included in any discussion of the risks of MC. Meatal stenosis may be recognized and diagnosed shortly after MC, or sometimes may be detected after several months or even years (Figs. 9.28 and 9.29).

Meatal stenosis is an under-recognized complication of circumcision in neonatal and nappy-aged boys. It is the most common serious complication of MC, and symptomatic presentation of meatal stenosis can be very late.[17]

Several circumcision techniques cause damage to the frenular branches of the dorsal penile artery, and it has been proposed that the resulting ischaemia of the meatus and, possibly, the distal part of the urethra may be responsible for meatal stenosis development in circumcised males. Investigations assessing the impact of frenular artery sparing circumcision techniques lend support to this theory. In one study, traditional infant circumcision preceded by ligation of the frenular artery was followed by meatal stenosis development in 15% of 105 boys during a mean follow-up period of 9 years; the corresponding proportion among 101 boys undergoing the same circumcision procedure but without initial ligation of the frenular artery was only 2%.[18]

In a review of 1009 circumcised boys who were examined after the age of 3 years, Van Howe[19] found an overall 2.8% incidence of symptomatic meatal stenosis after neonatal circumcision and it accounts for 26% of the late MC complications. The incidence of asymptomatic meatal stenosis (<5F meatal caliber) can be as high as 20%; however, its clinical significance is debatable.

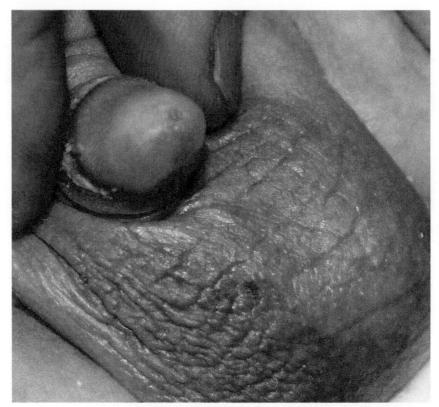

FIG. 9.28 Marked meatal stricture diagnosed a few weeks after male circumcision.

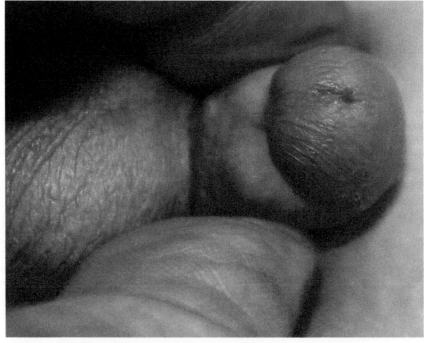

FIG. 9.29 Meatal stenosis discovered late after male circumcision.

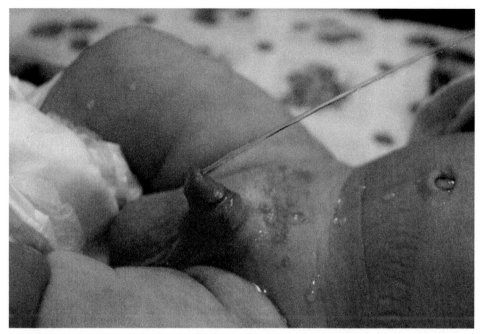

FIG. 9.30 Post-male circumcision meatal stenosis manifested with an upward deviated urinary stream, and an associated dermatitis in the suprapubic region is obvious.

For proper management and to avoid a medicolegal issue, it is mandatory for the physician to examine carefully, and sometimes to calibrate, the urinary meatus after preputial retraction and before committing MC to rule out not only the congenital cases of meatal stenosis but also other congenital anomalies such as an abnormally located meatus or an associated meatal dimple.

Meatal stenosis can lead to an upwardly deflected urinary stream, dysuria, urgency or difficulty with voiding and a flat uroflow curve (Fig. 9.30).

The diagnosis is readily made by inspection, and ventral meatotomy is the treatment. Following meatotomy, it is mandatory that the orifice be kept widely patent by periodic progressive dilatation with sound until such time as the calibre of the meatus remains generously large. Unrecognized or unfollowed cases after management may end with the sequel of lower urinary tract obstruction, such as chronic UTI, bladder trabeculations or even vesicoureteral reflux. In one Israeli study, 2 of the 14 (14%) boys with isolated meatal stenosis who had been circumcised in the neonatal period had radiographically confirmed vesicoureteral reflux.[20]

REFERENCES

1. Brook I. Infectious complications of circumcision and their prevention. *European Urology Focus.* 2016;2(Issue 4): 453–459.
2. Gee WF, Ansell JS. Neonatal circumcision: a ten year overview: with comparison of the Gomco clamp and the Plastibell device. *Pediatrics.* 1976;58(6):824–827.
3. Bliss DP, Healey PJ, Waldhausen JHT. Necrotizing fasciitis after Plastibell circumcision. *J Pediatr.* 1997;131(3): 459–462.
4. Bennett J, Breen C, Traverso H, Bano Agha S, Macia J, Boring J. Circumcision and neonatal tetanus: disclosure of risk and its reduction by topical antibiotics. *Int J Epidemiol.* 1999;28(2):263–266.
5. Williams N, Kapila L. Complications of circumcision. *Br J Surg.* 1993;80:1231.
6. Patel HI, Moriarty KP, Brisson PA, Feins NR. Genitourinary injuries in the newborn. *J Pediatr Surg.* 2001;36(1): 235–239.
7. Atikeler M, Onur R, Gecit I, Senol F, Cobanoglu B. Increased morbidity after circumcision from a hidden complication. *BJU Int.* 2001;88:938–940. https:// doi.org/10.1046/j.1464-4096.2001.02416.x.
8. Birley HDL, Walker MM, Ga L, et al. Clinical features and management of recurrent balanitis; association with recurrent washing. *Genitourin Med.* 1993;69:400–403.

9. David LM, Walzman M, Rajamanoharan S. Genital colonisation and infection with candida in heterosexual and homosexual males. *Genitourin Med.* 1997;73(5):394–396.

10. Pugliese J, Morey A, Peterson A. Lichen sclerosus: review of the literature and current recommendations for management. *J Urol.* 2007;178:2268e76.

11. Potter B. Balanitis xerotica obliterans manifesting on the stump of amputated penis. *Arch Dermatol.* 1959;79:473.

12. Bale PM, Lochhead A, Martin HC, Gollow I. Balanitis xerotica obliterans in children. *Pediatr Pathol.* 1987;7(5–6):617–627.

13. Thomas RM, Ridley CM, Black MM. The association of lichen sclerosus et atrophicus related disease in males. *Br J Dermatol.* 1983;109:661–664.

14. Zahorsky J. The ammoniacal diaper in infants and young children. *Am J Dis Child.* 1915;10:475.

15. von Bokay J. Sr.: *Gerhards Handbuch der Kinderheilkunde.* 1878;4:189.

16. Brennemann J. The ulcerated meatus in the circumcised child. *Am J Dis Child.* 1921;21:38–47.

17. Upadhyay V, Hammodat HM, Pease PW. Post circumcision meatal stenosis: 12 years' experience. *N Z Med J.* 1998;111(1060):57–58.

18. Kajbafzadeh AM, Kajbafzadeh M, Arbab M, Heidari F, Arshadi H, Milani SM. Post circumcision meatal stenosis in the neonates due to meatal devascularisation: a comparison of frenular artery sparing, Plastibell and conventional technique. *J Urol.* 2011;185:e132.

19. Van Howe RS. Variability in penile appearance and penile findings. *Br J Urol.* 1997;80:776–782.

20. Persad R, Sharma S, McTavish J, Imber C, Mouriquand PD. Clinical presentation and pathophysiology of meatal stenosis following circumcision. *Br J Urol.* 1995;75:91–93.

FURTHER READING

1. Escala JM, Rickwood AMK. Balanitis. *Br J Urol.* 1989;63:196–197.

CHAPTER 10

Nonaesthetic Circumcision Scarring

MOHAMED A BAKY FAHMY, MD, FRCS

ABSTRACT

Circumcision may be undertaken as a body modification of the genitals to change the look of the penis to appeal more to certain aesthetics, but sometimes it may leave a permanent change of the natal characteristics of a body part, which will ever be subject to dispute, particularly from the cosmetic point of view. Many complications may result after nonaesthetic preputial cutting or the unhealthy healing of the circumcision wound. These complications usually manifest late, weeks or months after the procedure, and result in early family dissatisfaction and later on have a psychic impact on a man's satisfaction with his penis and may lead to loss of self-esteem.

KEYWORDS

Incomplete circumcision; Keloid and hypertrophic scar; Paraphimosis; Penile adhesions; Phimosis; Post-circumcision lymphoedema; Post-MC concealed penis; Post-MC smegma collections; Residual prepuce; Skin bridge; Sutures marks; Untidy circumcision.

Circumcision may be undertaken as a body modification of the genitals to change the look of the penis to appeal more to certain aesthetics, but sometimes it may leave a permanent change of the natal characteristics of a body part, which will ever be subject to dispute, particularly from the cosmetic point of view.

Many complications may result after nonaesthetic preputial cutting or the unhealthy healing of the circumcision wound. These complications usually manifest late, weeks or months after the procedure, and result in early family dissatisfaction and later on have a psychic impact on a man's satisfaction with his penis and may lead to loss of self-esteem.

Complications of excessive or improper tissue scarring after male circumcision (MC) have a wide spectrum of presentations, not only including aesthetic problems, but also a functional drawbacks could also result. These complications have variable incidence and are not commonly reported, and they are difficult to classify, as many categories overlap each other or occur in sequence, for example, incomplete MC may result in cicatricial phimosis and excess inner preputial layer which may result in a keloid scar. Some complications may be termed as incomplete circumcision by some surgeons, but it is called untidy circumcision by others.

There are no definite universal criteria for the ideal circumcision scar, and also circumcision is not performed in the same manner in different communities. A 'normal' looking circumcised penis in a country may seem ugly and unacceptable by people from other parts of the world.

Generally, the circumcision line should be close to the glans as possible, limiting the width of inner prepuce up to 5—6 mm in newborns and 7—8 mm in older boys; this not only helps give an acceptable look to the penis but also prevents the so-called 'entrapped penis' by making it impossible for the circumcision line to move distal to the glans and retract proximally easily[1] (Fig. 10.1).

Post-MC aesthetic complications are mostly iatrogenic and imminent, and certain factors may be considered as leading to poor cosmesis, such as

- Impertinent tissue handling.
- Insufficient haemostasis.
- Using thick heavy sutures with long absorption time.
- Failing to recognize anatomic diversities or abnormalities.
- Excessive resection of prepuce.
- Too tight dressing.

There is no study documenting the penile appearance beyond the first year of life in the circumcised population, but it is estimated that at least 2.8% of parents will complain of the cosmetic appearance.[1]

We will discuss nonaesthetic circumcision scarring complications under the following headings:

- Untidy circumcision
- Penile adhesions
- Skin bridge
- Incomplete circumcision
- Post-MC concealed penis (CP)
- Phimosis
- Paraphimosis
- Keloid and hypertrophic scar

Complications in Male Circumcision. https://doi.org/10.1016/B978-0-323-68127-8.00010-7

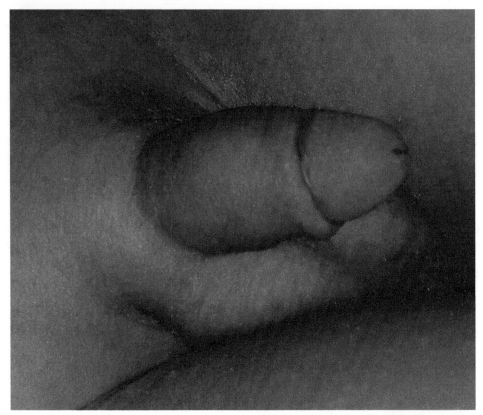

FIG. 10.1 An aesthetic regular scar with a minimal rim of inner prepuce after sleeve circumcision.

- Suture marks
- Post-MC smegma collections
- Post-circumcision lymphoedema

UNTIDY CIRCUMCISION (UGLY CIRCUMCISION SCAR)

Circumcision is a procedure that will alter the entire anatomy and the look of the penis, which itself carries a countless variations among populations, so it is extremely difficult to standardize the shape and appearance of the penis after this operation. Different studies concluded with a diverse opinion about the aesthetic look of the penis after MC.[1]

Cosmetic results were compared and rated by the Patient and Observer Scar Assessment Scale (POSAS)[2] as the following:

Good: Linear scar with minimal or no puckering.
Average: Linear scar with puckering of the surrounding skin without depression.
Poor: Severe puckering and depressed irregular scar.

Fig. 10.1 represents my own opinion about the desirable scar after circumcision by dissection method, with a thin circular scar around the coronal sulcus with a narrow rim of inner prepuce left, a preserved frenulum and adequate penile skin to allow, later on, the erected penis to stretch smoothly.

Irregularity of the healed wound after MC, which may result in an untidy scar, is usually due to heavy suturing, post-MC infection, haematoma formation or leaving the compression bandage for a longer time after circumcision. Such cases are different from cases of incomplete circumcision, which had a normal scar edge but excess amount of residual prepuce, and also cases of localized skin bridges.[3]

Excessive scarring at the circumcision edge may be due to uneven incision lines, which usually occur in guillotine method and free-handed sleeve circumcision by unexperienced surgeons. Such cases may deserve correction and proper reconstruction under general anaesthesia by a reconstructive surgeon with a good experience in penile surgery, as any attempt to repair such cases early by an inexperienced surgeon may result

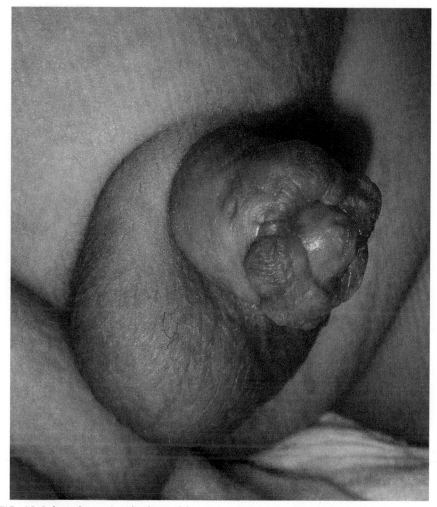

FIG. 10.2 Irregular post-male circumcision wavy scar covering the sulcus and part of the glans.

in more skin loss, penile concealment and deformities (Fig. 10.2).

Unequally inner or outer preputial cutting may result in excess skin or mucous membrane in one side of the healed scar. This may be encountered in either free-handed or guillotine method, but uncommon with the use of the Gomco and Plastibell methods (Figs. 10.3 and 10.4).

Bad mucosal healing, irregular circumcision scar and suture sinus tracts result collectively in a bad cosmesis of the scarring around the corneal sulcus (Fig. 10.5).

Glans injury or cauterization by diathermy during MC, or a post-circumcision infection, may result in isolated scarring and disfigurement of the glans penis, and such cases are extremely difficult to repair (Fig. 10.6).

The whole concept of an aesthetic prepuce will be discussed in Chapter 11.

PENILE ADHESIONS

Penile adhesion is a broad term for different pathologic condition. The most common one is the localized form of skin bridge. Penile adhesions are a relatively common complication of circumcision, especially at neonatal age, and are the primary reasons for reoperation in the late postoperative period.

Predisposing Factors

Adhesions are more likely in children with an increased weight for length percentile, in children with a large suprapubic fat pad with abnormal dartos attachments to the skin and in cases of pre-existing penoscrotal webbing or ventral penile skin deficiency. Adhesions are also common in neonatal MC, as the inner prepuce

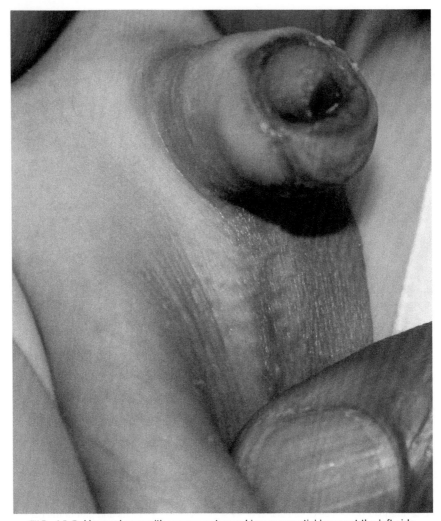

FIG. 10.3 Unequal scar with excess outer and inner preputial layers at the left side.

is physiologically adherent to the glans, and any forcible attempt to separate it will result in a denuded glandular surface, which will easily heal with fibrous scarring with the surrounding penile skin. Different forms of penile adhesions may follow post-MC infectious complications, especially bacterial balanitis; also, balanitis xerotica obliterans (BXO) cases after MC may be associated or complicated with severe penile adhesions, especially if the circumcision wound is untidy (Fig. 10.7).

Adhesions could be seen at different levels and between different parts of the penis:

- Adhesions between excess remnants of mucous membrane (inner preputial layer) and the glans penis, which may be partial or complete forming a ring around the glans (Fig. 10.8).
- Complete adhesions of the redundant cut edges of the prepuce with the raw surface of the glans, which may eventually lead to cicatricial phimosis (Fig. 10.9).
- Adhesions between a localized raw surface of the glans and penile skin forming different forms of skin bridging between the penile shaft and the glans penis, crossing the coronal sulcus (Fig. 10.10).

All these adhesions of the mucosal collar to the glans are avoidable by gentle preputial retraction, meticulous tissue handling and use of barrier ointments in the early post-operative period.

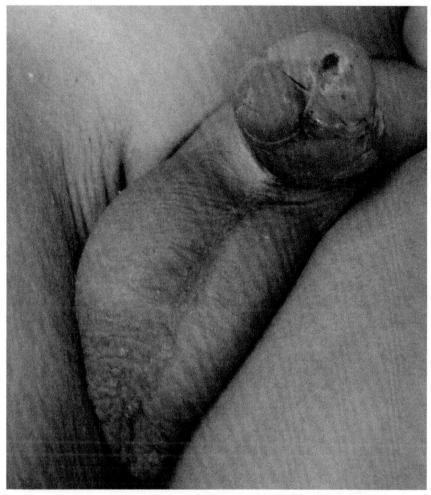

FIG. 10.4 An excess inner preputial layer at the right side of the glans.

SKIN BRIDGES

Sometimes a localized area of adhesion results in the formation of well-formed excess skin bridges between the skin of the penile shaft and the glans penis (Fig. 10.10). These epithelialized adhesions can lead to penile chordee, torsion, and later on, it may result in a painful erection due to tethering of the erected penis. Skin bridges in the ventral penile surface are usually more symptomatic than the dorsal and lateral ones. The abnormal scarring will also make the circumcised penis looks ugly with an obvious disfigurement (Fig. 10.11).

Smegma often accumulates under those skin bridges, and it may form a well-capsulated cyst (Fig. 10.12).

Skin bridges could be seen as a single area of wedge like skin creeping over the glans with different sizes at one side, or multiple scars of different shapes around the glans (Figs. 10.13 and 10.14).

Excess redundant skin after circumcision, physiologic retraction of the penis due to a suprapubic fat pad and diaper irritation of the penis may be predisposing factors.

Incidence

How such this problems arise is not completely clear, as true incidence is difficult to estimate. But some authors reported that skin bridges accounted for nearly 30% of the late complications. The rate of complications usually decreases with age, owing to the epithelial separation of the adhesions (71% of infants, 28% of 1–5 year old children, 8% of 1–9 year old children and 2% of children older than 9 years).[4]

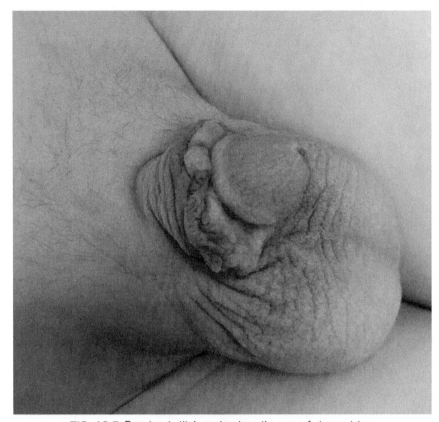

FIG. 10.5 Prominent stitch marks along the scar of circumcision.

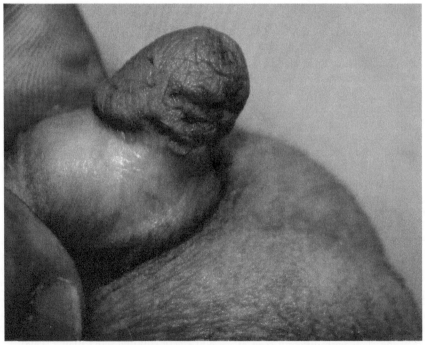

FIG. 10.6 Multiple glandular injuries leading to disfigurement.

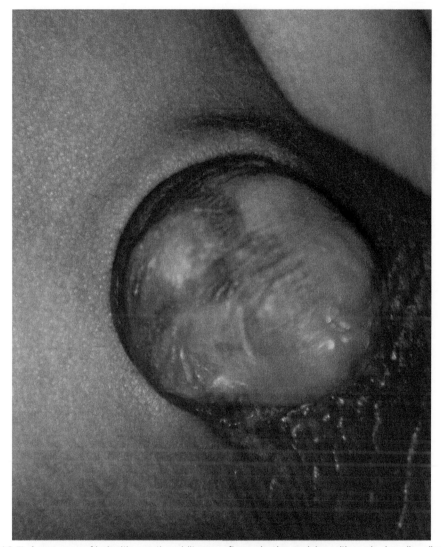

FIG. 10.7 A rare case of balanitis xerotica obliterans after male circumcision with marked penile adhesions.

Treatment

This complication could be avoided by completely freeing the inner preputial layer from the glans at the time of circumcision; also, if any glanular abrasions, injury or ulcer is detected during MC, it should be dressed and managed properly until complete healing to avoid the natural cohesion between the denuded area of the glans and the penile skin. Use of low-dose corticosteroids has been relatively unsuccessful in lysing these well-formed adhesions. The adhesions can be excised in the office with the application of local anaesthesia or in the operating room with the use of general or regional anaesthesia by suturing the glandular and shaft defects with fine absorbable sutures (Fig. 10.15).

In my opinion, routine suturing of both preputial layers with fine stitches either continuously or with interruptions, even in neonatal MC, will protect the healing incision from such complications.

INCOMPLETE CIRCUMCISION

Nomenclature: Residual prepuce, inadequate circumcision or excess foreskin.

The high degree of variability in the appearance of penis after MC could not be related to the technique

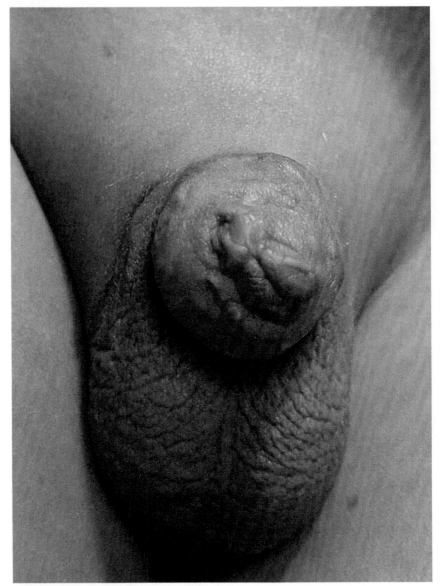

FIG. 10.8 Extensive penile adhesion between the circumcision scar and the glans, forming a ring around the glans, with marked disfigurement.

used or to the physician using it. When operating on an infantile penis, the surgeon cannot adequately judge the appropriate amount of tissue to remove because the penis will change considerably as the child ages, such that a small difference at the time of surgery may translate into a large difference in the adult circumcised penis. Any one dealing with penile anomalies can recognize the diversity and wide variation in the normal anatomy of different penile structures because many neonates may have a very long prepuce, which is called 'akroposthia', and some may have a deficient prepuce, with an exposed distal glans without preputial retraction, so the amount of prepuce to be removed in MC should be tailored for each baby according to the length of his prepuce. This is extremely difficult to achieve in mass circumcision or even in a hospital with a high

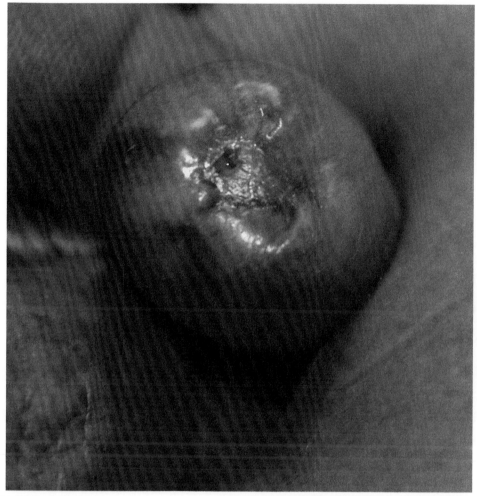

FIG. 10.9 Penile adhesions forming a scar ring with the glans around the urinary meatus, which may result in cicatricial phimosis.

number of cases. To date, there have been no published studies showing the ability of a circumciser to predict the later appearance of the penis.[5]

According to the previous studies, between 1% and 9.5% of boys circumcised at birth will have the procedure revised or redone and 2.8% of parents will complain of the cosmetic appearance.[3]

Leaving a short inner prepuce is achievable in open sleeve and clamp techniques (Gomco and others), but it is not possible in the traditional guillotine-type circumcision, which leaves a very long inner prepuce with a circumcision line placed in almost the middle of the penile shaft (Fig. 10.16). Unfortunately, this is still the most common technique performed by nonmedical personnel in large parts of the world.

The inner foreskin and outer foreskin are a separate entities, and not the opposite sides of a single layer of tissue. They are not attached to each other and in consequence are mobile with respect to each other. Thus it is possible to remove unequal amounts of the two layers. Understanding this point is crucial for recognition of a different circumcision styles.

If we can exclude other complications, the penile looks after different techniques of MC may be one of these two common styles:
- MC style that retained the inner foreskin (the 'high' style): The circumcision scar line of a man with the high style will be partway up his penis (Fig. 10.16). If the scar is moving freely without tightness, it is called high loose, otherwise it is a high tight one. Of course,

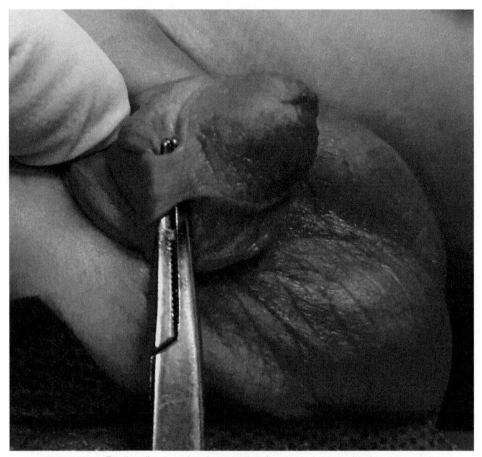

FIG. 10.10 Penile adhesions forming a well-defined skin bridge with the glans penis.

these cases should be differentiated from cases of sever skin loss, which may heal with intense fibrosis.

- MC style that removed the inner foreskin (the 'low' style): The circumcision scar line of a man with the low style will be close to the rim of his glans (Fig. 10.17). If the scar ring is tight, it may be problematic and may be considered as a concealed penis(CP) or even an acquired phimosis. A loose scar is an acceptable form, but it may be an indication for MC redo according to some parents' wishes. So the circumcised scar could be classified as
- High loose
- High tight
- Low loose
- Low tight

The amount of penile skin excised can also lead to many other complications, as insufficient or asymmetric prepuce excision can result in a cosmetic and social dilemma for the parents and the child, especially when the child gets older (Fig. 10.2).

A circumcision that is too loose may not leave the glans completely uncovered but it will, in other words, be a partial circumcision, and this is not in itself a problem but it may not meet parental or religious expectations. However, there is one important exception, if the scar can mobilize in front of the corona then it will shrink and create secondary phimosis, which requires recircumcision. If a partial circumcision is deliberately chosen then the best approach is to remove the inner foreskin completely, so that the scar will be in the sulcus. At puberty the penis will usually outgrow the skin and leave the glans exposed, as the degree of skin covering the glans after neonatal circumcision peaks at 6 months of age.

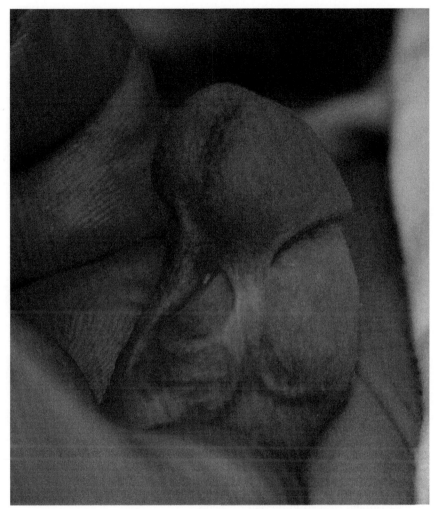

FIG. 10.11 A ventral skin bridge results in penile curvature during erection.

Management

Unlike neonatal circumcision, circumcision revision requires general anaesthesia, for which several techniques have been described. Excessive skin excision can result in penile chordee, torsion and lateral deviation. These conditions, if necessary to repair, may require penile skin flaps or Z-plasty for closure.

Excessive skin removal can also result in a trapped penis from a cicatricial scar. The trapped penis can be managed with betamethasone conservatively, vertical relaxation incision and then a formal repair. The use of 0.05% betamethasone in conjunction with manual retraction in children with a trapped penis due to a dense cicatrix of the residual foreskin distal to the glans has a 79% success in softening the cicatrix with easy exposure of the glans or mild persistence of the cicatrix amenable to vertical relaxation incision.[5]

While many people favour retaining a lot of inner foreskin, this can sometimes cause problems. The inner skin is very thin and stretchable, and if there happens to be a lot of postoperative swelling, it can permanently stretch the skin, leaving it loose and puffy. This has no effect on penile function, but it can appear unsightly (Fig. 10.18).

If the physician succeeds to convince the parents (or sometimes the circumcised adult) not to revise the circumcision in cases of low or incomplete MC, special attention should be paid to the retained part of the prepuce. Generally, the circumcised penis requires more care than the intact penis, especially during the first

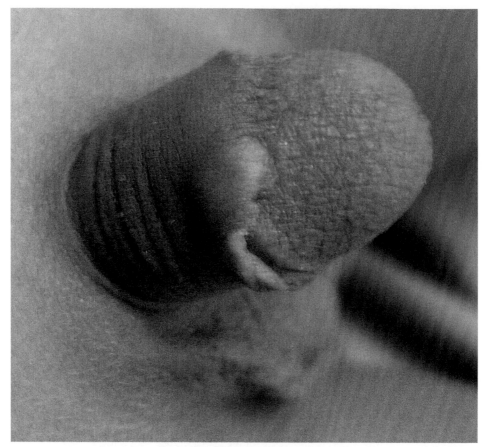

FIG. 10.12 A small smegma cyst formed under a skin bridge.

3 years of life; any skin covering the glans in circumcised boys should be retracted and cleaned to prevent adhesions and debris accumulation.

In contrast to the general belief that smegma is not present, or at least not accumulated, in circumcised boys, we encountered many circumcised babies with the same smegma accumulation and configuration as in the intact ones, especially in those children with low loose type of circumcision. So all the adverse effects of smegma will be seen in an adult with a retained long prepuce after circumcision (Fig. 10.19).

POST-MALE CIRCUMCISION CONCEALED PENIS

Generally, CP refers to an anomaly such that the penis appears to be short, even though its length is normal. CP may be divided into three groups according to the Maizels classification, which is based on the aetiologic mechanism: buried penis, webbed penis and trapped penis.[67]

One or more mechanisms may contribute to concealment in each case:

- Buried penis describes a condition in which a penis remains under the level of pubic skin because of the excessive suprapubic fat or the loose attachment of penile skin to the dartos.
- Webbed penis is a condition in which there is extra skin between the scrotal raphe and distal penis, obscuring the penoscrotal angle.
- Trapped penis refers to a condition in which a normal penis is depressed under the skin following a surgical procedure, generally circumcision, and looks concealed, and this type is our main concern herein (Fig. 10.20).

Williams et al. reported a rate of 9% CP among those applying for routine circumcision. The same study reported a 63% incidence of CP among those applying

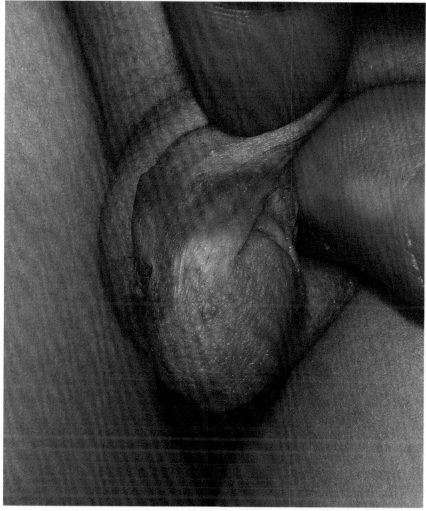

FIG. 10.13 A wide area of skin creeping over the glans.

for circumcision revision (26% trapped penis and 37% insufficient circumcision).[8] It is possible that one may refrain from excising sufficient prepuce in order to avoid a more complicated picture in a case with partial CP and as a result insufficient circumcision may take place. In a baby with CP, generous excision of the penile skin in an effort to make the penis visible usually leads to a crippled problem of trapped penis, with almost no local penile skin surrounding the penis, which will require flaps or grafts for correction.

This complication is commonly seen in overweight children or in those with extensive suprapubic fat and is expected to associate cases of microphallus and webbed penis.

Post-MC CPs could be classified into complete and partial concealment.

Complete

This is commonly seen in neonatal circumcision in which the penis is completely hidden and covered by either the scarred penile skin or the scarred preputial remnants (Fig. 10.20).

Partial

In this condition, the glans penis is visible but the penile shaft is partially covered by the scarred skin, and this is usually seen in older children (Fig. 10.21).

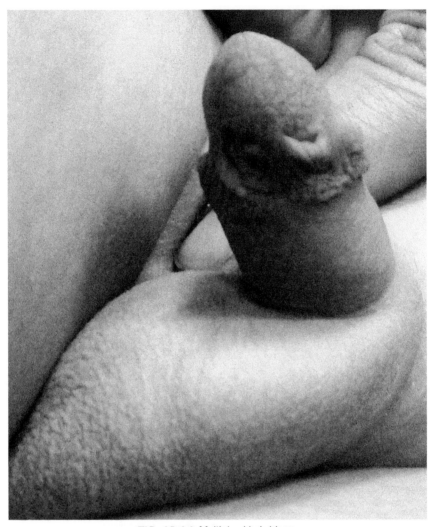

FIG. 10.14 Multiple skin bridges.

Penile entrapment by the circumcision scar may be complicated by an ascending urinary tract infection (UTI), balanitis and may lead to a cicatricial phimosis.

In children with a secondary CP, but without phimosis, observation may be an option, as the cosmetic appearance tends to improve with age and surgery should be delayed until the child is at least 3 years of age. Borsellino et al.[9] reported that a staged revision surgery was required in a majority of their cases because the penile shaft skin was also excised along with the prepuce.

POST-MALE CIRCUMCISION PHIMOSIS

Nomenclature: Cicatricial phimosis, acquired phimosis, preputial stenosis.

Post-MC phimosis is a sort of penile adhesion, with extensive scarring distal to the urinary meatus, covering the glans penis completely with inability to retract the preputial remnants proximally (Fig. 10.22).

When operating on the infantile penis, the surgeon cannot adequately judge the appropriate amount of tissue to remove because the penis will change considerably as the child ages, such that a small difference at

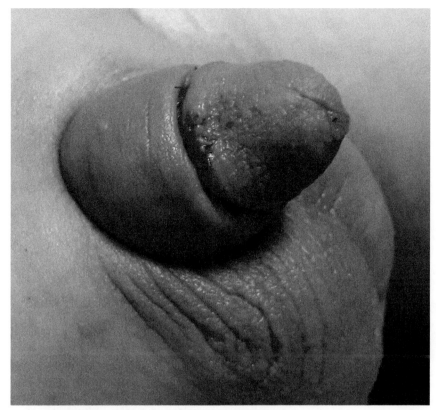

FIG. 10.15 Surgically excised skin bridges, and fine stitching of the preputial and glandular defects.

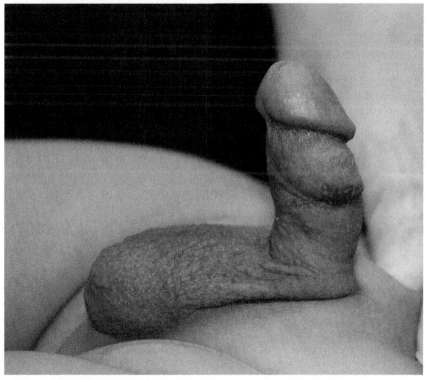

FIG. 10.16 High loose male circumcision with excess inner prepuce.

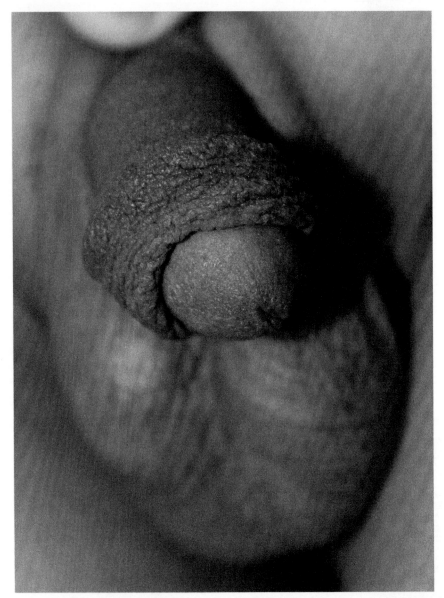

FIG. 10.17 Low loose male circumcision with excess of both the preputial layers, but without constriction.

the time of surgery may translate into a large difference in the adult circumcised penis. Phimosis with a trapped penis is an infrequent but important complication of circumcision. This condition is more likely to occur in older infants and those with poor attachment of the penile skin to the shaft.

Incidences of 0.32%, 0.4% and 1% have been reported for preputial stenosis resulting from neonatal circumcision. Although the exact incidence of preputial stenosis (phimosis) in boys with intact penis is unknown, it is most likely between 0.9% and 1.9%.[10]

Penile inflammation (balanitis) may be more common in circumcised boys with preputial stenosis than in uncircumcised children with phimosis. The common finding of subpreputial debris in circumcised infants may reflect inadequate hygiene; these debris usually consisted of lint, dirt, talcum powder, stool and detritus. The association between subpreputial debris

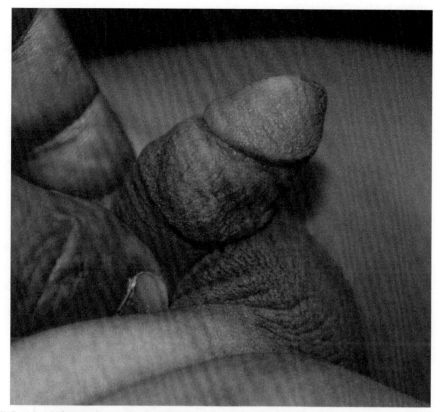

FIG. 10.18 Incomplete male circumcision, with a long inner prepuce, looks puffy and inflamed.

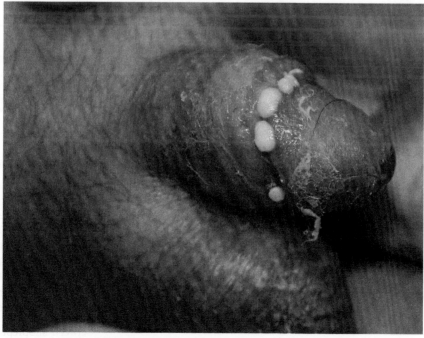

FIG. 10.19 A smegma collection with dirt in a circumcised boy.

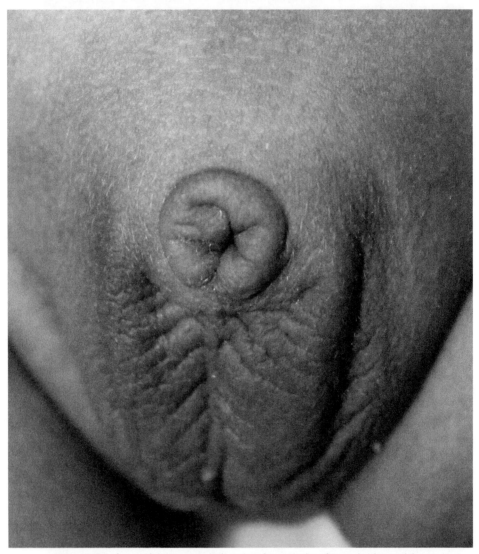

FIG. 10.20 A completely concealed penis a few months after male circumcision.

and coronal adhesions implicates poor hygiene as a possible cause. In the normal penis, muscle fibres are arranged in a whorl to form a sphincter that keeps unwanted contaminants out. Urine swirling under the prepuce in a normal infant before expulsion flushes any contaminants from the subpreputial space and may explain the paucity of findings in this population. Subpreputial debris may have been under-reported in young boys with intact penis because forcible retraction of the foreskin, which is a harmful practice, was not frequently performed.[10] Difficult micturition is a common symptom, and UTI and even urinary retention may complicate the case (Fig. 10.23).

Treatment

Unlike the treatment of primary phimosis, application of local corticosteroid cream does not cause separation of secondary glanular adhesions after circumcision.[11] Early recognition allows outpatient treatment with excellent results, avoiding operative intervention with general anaesthesia, by genital separation of the scarred tissue from the glans and widening of the stenosed hiatus.

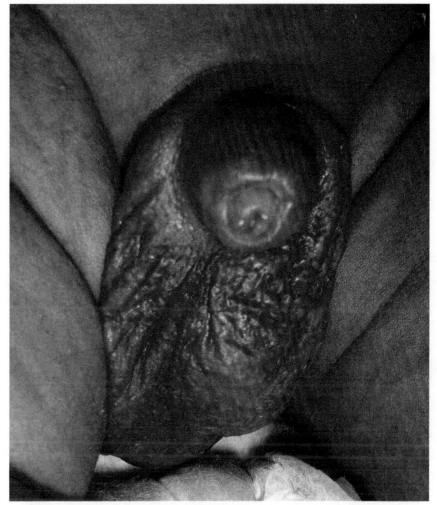

FIG. 10.21 A partially concealed penis with only visible glans penis.

In difficult and neglected cases, repair is scheduled electively under general anaesthesia and is best started by marking the part of skin to be removed precisely and a proximal incision applied, removing the redundant skin and preputial membrane as separate layers starting from up and going down to the meatus. But great caution should be exerted to avoid excessive skin removal, and the technique can be accomplished by fine stitching of the penile skin with the internal preputial remnant rim (Figs. 10.24 and 10.25).

A special entity may be encountered in adults suffering from BXO who were managed by circumcision as a treatment modality. As a few cases may develop cicatricial phimosis if the prepuce is removed incompletely and balanitis recurs, adhesions between the glans and the prepuce are also common and these adhesions are difficult or impossible to separate. Such cases could be managed by leaving a fine layer of dartos covering the glans rather than denuding it, and the residual epithelial cells in this layer are left to recover the glans over the following weeks.[12]

PARAPHIMOSIS

Paraphimosis is a true urologic emergency that occurs in uncircumcised men when the foreskin becomes trapped behind the corona of the glans penis, which can lead to strangulation of the glans as well as painful vascular compromise, distal venous engorgement, oedema and even glandular necrosis. Phimosis, by comparison, is

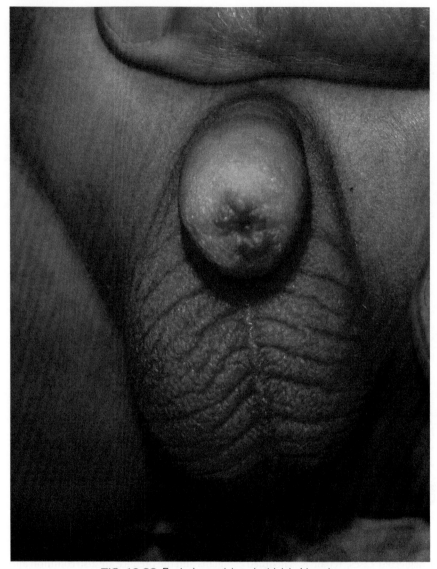

FIG. 10.22 Post-circumcision cicatricial phimosis.

the condition in which the foreskin is unable to be retracted behind the glans penis (Fig. 10.26).

Paraphimosis could happen because boys have been encouraged to retract the foreskin for physiologic phimosis by parents or medical staff.

Paraphimosis commonly occurs iatrogenically when the foreskin is retracted for cleaning, for placement of a urinary catheter, during a procedure such as cystoscopy or during penile examination. Iatrogenic paraphimosis is an acute complication of MC in neonates and children when the circumciser fails to reposition the prepuce after initial retraction during the procedure. This complication is not related to the aesthetic complication but is discussed herein for its relation to phimosis.

Incidence

In uncircumcised children, aged 4 months to 12 years, with foreskin problems, paraphimosis (0.2%) is less common than other penile disorders such as balanitis (5.9%), irritation (3.6%), penile adhesions (1.5%) and phimosis (2.6%).[13]

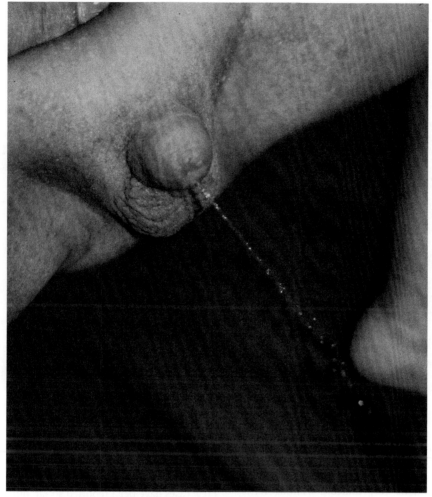

FIG. 10.23 Difficulty in micturition with acquired phimosis.

There is no estimation of the incidence of paraphimosis, which complicates the procedure of MC, but we dealt with many cases referred from the primary care centres with a strangulated preputial hiatus behind the coronal sulcus after different procedures of circumcision.

Factors that may predispose to paraphimosis include the following:
- Forcible retraction of prepuce, while the baby had different grades of phimosis.
- Babies with congenitally tight preputial opening without inflammation.
- Neonatal circumcision by inexperienced personnel.
- It is not a rare complication during circumcision of children with blood-related diseases (Fig. 10.27).
- Paraphimosis caused by dislodgement of the plastic ring represents 41.8% of complications among children circumcised by the Plastibell technique, a complication that was responsible for the highest rate of reoperation.[14]

Sequelae

Paraphimosis encountered during routine MC is a controllable complication and easy to be managed without any sequel, if treated immediately or referred to specialized centres. But glans penis ischaemia or necrosis caused by paraphimosis is a rare complication of a urologic emergency, with a few cases were reported in the literature.[15]

Management

In most instances, manual compression can reduce the preputial oedema within the first few hours; however,

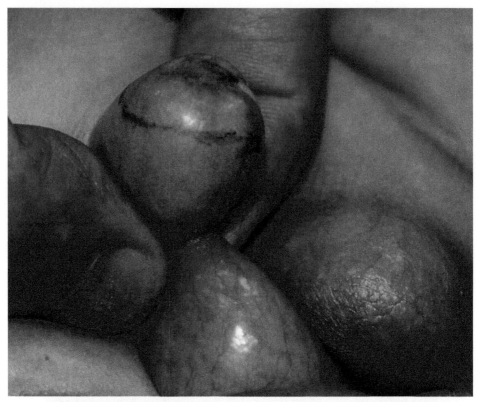

FIG. 10.24 Marking the proposed incision before correction of cicatricial phimosis.

enthusiastic attempts without adequate analgesia and sedation should be avoided, as they are distressing, are likely to fail and may make further examination or treatment interventions very difficult. Various techniques are described to treat this condition, including applying granulated sugar to the penis, adding multiple punctures to the oedematous foreskin before compression, injecting hyaluronidase beneath the narrow band to release it and wrapping the distal penis in a saline-solution-soaked gauze swab and squeezing gently but firmly for 5–10 min. Thereafter, physicians are supposed to push forcefully on the glans with the thumbs, while pulling the foreskin with the fingers. However, an emergency dorsal slit may be necessary in late cases. Generally, some authors advise completion of circumcision for paraphimosis, whereas others insist that circumcision is not advisable and could be postponed or deferred as the foreskin is oedematous and other major injuries may supervene.[16]

KELOID FORMATION

Since Warwick and Dickson[17] firstly described their experiences with a post-circumcision keloid in 1993, only a few cases have been reported so far, but it is expected that many cases may escape proper diagnosis and reporting.

Keloids are benign, hyperproliferative scar tissue growths characterized by excessive deposition of collagen and other extracellular matrix components.

Although the exact pathogenetic mechanisms are still unknown, extracellular matrix abnormalities, aberrant collagen turnover, mechanical tension and genetic immune dysfunction have all been proposed as pathogenetic hypotheses. In addition, fibroblast cells derived from keloid tissue display an increased proliferation and density, among many other characteristics.

The most likely cause of post-MC keloid was the postoperative dehiscence resulting in prolonged wound healing in a genetically predisposed individual.

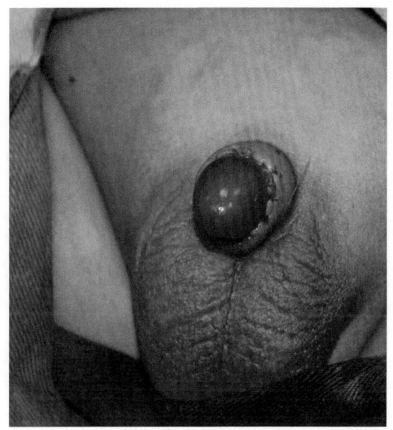

FIG. 10.25 After removing the excess constricting skin in cicatricial phimosis, fine absorbable stitches are applied.

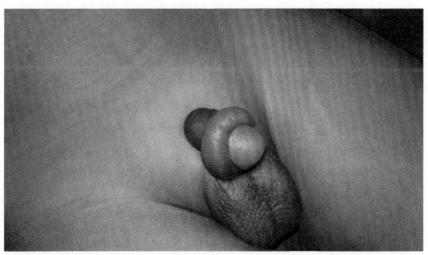

FIG. 10.26 A case of paraphimosis with an oedematous constricted prepuce behind the coronal sulcus.

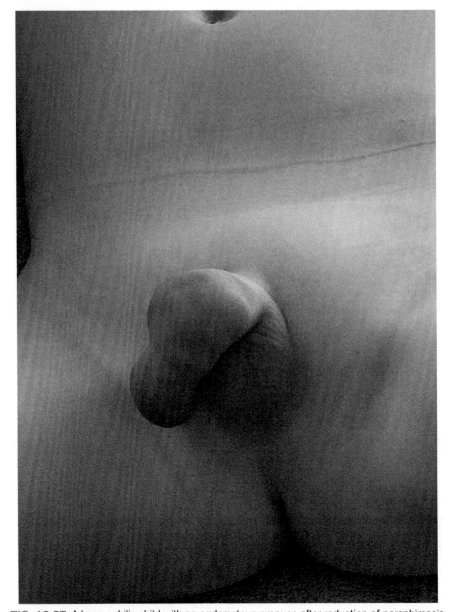

FIG. 10.27 A haemophilic child with an oedematous prepuce after reduction of paraphimosis.

Although keloid formation has been documented to be most frequent in patients between the ages of 15 and 45 years, only a few cases were reported below 12 years of age.[18]

Clinically a keloid is an abnormal development consisting of a raised, firm, thickened, red piece of scar tissue. Such abnormal scar at the site of circumcision creates a grotesque deformation of the organ, with obstruction of its function. Different forms of keloid, either localized or circumferential, had been reported after MC (Fig. 10.28).

Like other keloids of the body, the post-MC keloid seems to be more common in the black races. The predisposing factors are prolonged wound healing, foreign body implant during circumcision and rough manipulation of the delicate penile skin.

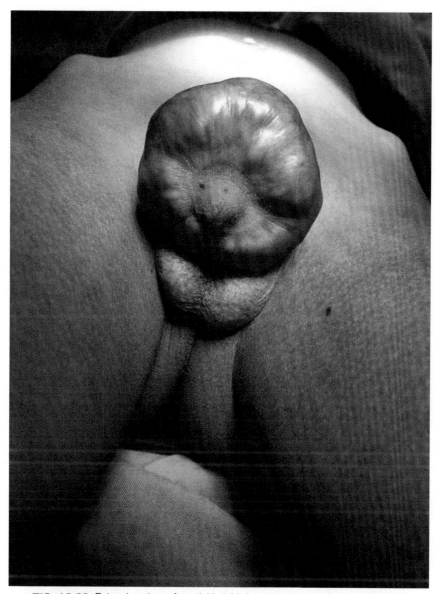

FIG. 10.28 Extensive circumferential keloid developed at the circumcision scar.

Less extensive prominent scars can occur with severe fibrosis around the coronal sulcus, and mild forms of hypertrophic scar of the healing wound after circumcision are not rare, but uncommonly reported. We diagnosed a few cases with a localized area of hypertrophic scar, especially in older children; such cases may respond to prolonged use of a potent corticosteroid, without a need for surgical intervention (Fig. 10.29).

Keloid excision with or without skin grafting is indicated as a different postoperative measure to avoid recurrence of a keloid tissue. Radiation therapy is contraindicated in children and is not desirable for penile keloids because of the close proximity of germ cells. Intralesional corticosteroid injection decreases fibroblast proliferation, collagen synthesis and suppresses pro-inflammatory mediators. The most commonly

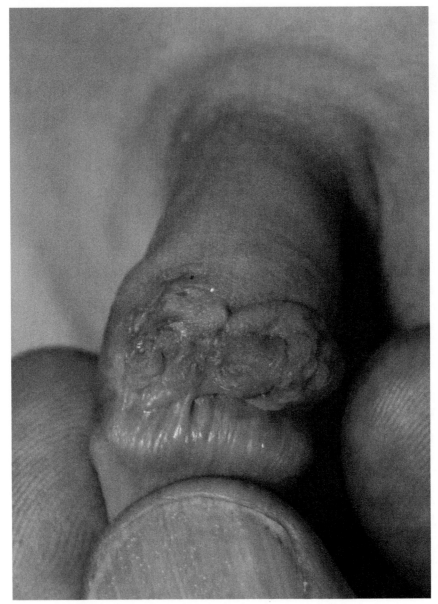

FIG. 10.29 A localized hypertrophic scar after circumcision.

used drug for steroid injection is triamcinolone aceto-
nide suspension at a dose of 5–10 mg/mL, which is
injected intralesionally.[19]

SUTURE MARKS

Post-MC suture marks are sometimes termed as spitting
sutures, which are detected weeks to months after surgery if the body rejects the sutures (again, from the

stitches not absorbed as intended) and attempts to
remove them by pushing the stitches out to the surface
of the skin. Sutures that migrate in this way have been
known to be the source of additional problems, such
as a penile disfigurement from the untidy stitches marks
or fibrosis (Fig. 10.5).

It is recommended for skin closure after MC to be
done with the most delicate rapidly absorbable sutures.
As the inner foreskin of newborns and infants is fragile,

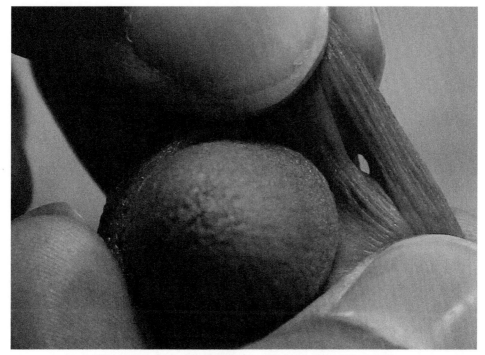

FIG. 10.30 A case of small stitch sinus in the preputial remnant.

6/0 or 7/0 quickly absorbable materials such as poly-glactin or polyglecaprone can be used. For older kids and adults, 5/0 quickly absorbable materials may be used. Using medical cyanoacrylate is a good alternative to stitching. It avoids permanent suture marks and suture tunnels that may be problematic. Meticulous haemostasis is vital before cyanoacrylate application. Subcuticular (separate or continuous) suturing, which has similar advantages, can also be used by giving some more time and effort.

Thick and slowly absorbable materials cause permanent suture tracts, which are a common sequel, resulting in disfigurement of the MC scar; very rarely small sinuses may be encountered long time after circumcision at the site of nonabsorbable stitches (Fig. 10.30).

A small stitch granuloma with or without smegma collection may also be seen with the stitch remnants (Fig. 10.31).

POST-MALE CIRCUMCISION SMEGMA COLLECTION

Definition: The word smegma is of Greek origin meaning soap or an ointment.

Smegmoma: Preputial smegma cyst.

Smegmaliths: Pieces of hard contaminated and retained smegma.

Smegma has a characteristic slimy odour and is composed of epithelial debris, fat and proteins. It has mixed bacterial flora, including the smegma bacillus (*Mycobacterium smegmatis*) in 50% of man.

Smegma is the natural secretion of the prepuce, like other body secretions, such as earwax. So it is not harmful by itself, unless it is complicated by other pathogens, bacterial colonization, viral overgrowth or a combination of organisms. Smegma collection is usually associated with phimosis and different forms of balanitis or balanoposthitis.

Smegma secretion and distribution had a great variation between individuals and between different ages without a clear explanation. Wright[20] states that smegma is produced from minute microscopic protrusions of the mucosal surface of the foreskin and that living cells constantly grow towards the surface, undergo fatty degeneration, separate off and form smegma.

Smegma should be cleaned frequently in uncircumcised boys by the mother during childhood and by the boy himself later on. Circumcised boys, especially those with excess skin remnants, may have a marked smegma

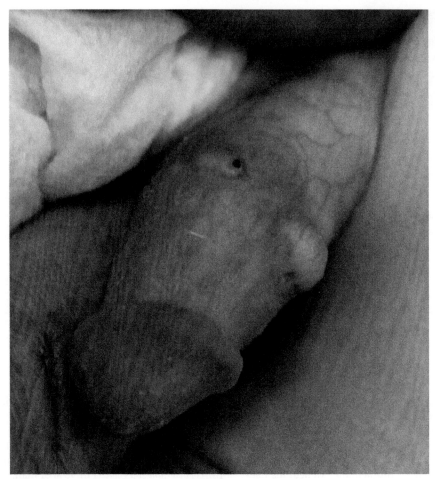

FIG. 10.31 Multiple small collections of granulation tissue around a nonabsorbable stitch, with smegma collection.

secretion and attention should be paid to clean it as in uncircumcised boys (Fig. 10.19).

During circumcision, smegma should be cleaned and removed meticulously with saline wash, otherwise any retained small pieces will be entrapped and will accumulate between the edges of the incised prepuce and result in different forms of cysts of smegma, which may become large and will lead to different complications.

Smegma Cyst

Aggregation of smegma in circumcised children is not rare and may present alone without any other complications or in association with skin bridges (Fig. 10.12) or with stitch granuloma (Fig. 10.31) as a yellowish cystic or doughy swelling of different sizes at the cut edges of the prepuce (Fig. 10.32). Sometimes the swelling may become larger, disfiguring the penis (Fig. 10.33). It is

usually presented as a single swelling, but cases with multiple small cysts are not rare (Fig. 10.34).

Smegma, produced under the foreskin, is made of 27% fat and 13% protein and contributes to the higher occurrence of *Malassezia* fungal species in uncircumcised versus circumcised men (49% vs. 7%). The frequency of yeast colonization in smegma is around 11%.[21]

It is considered as an inclusion cyst, and if seen at the ventral surface of the penis, or along the median raphe, it should be differentiated from other rare true penile cysts, such as parameatal cysts, mucoid cysts or median raphe cysts[22] (Fig. 10.35).

These cysts are liable to irritation, traumatic rupture and infection with abscess formation. This complication is avoidable, but once diagnosed, careful excision under general or regional anaesthesia, with meticulous penile skin closure, is indicated and will avoid recurrence.[23]

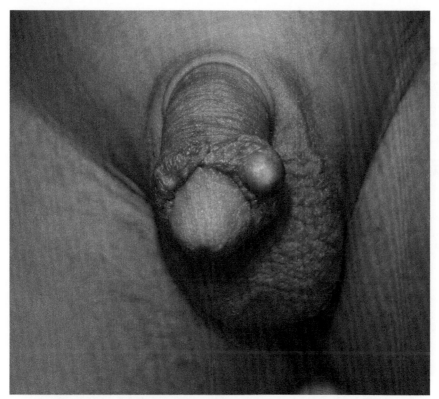

FIG. 10.32 A single small smegma cyst at the rim of a circumcision scar.

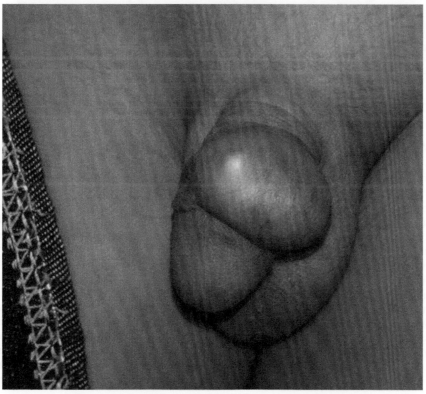

FIG. 10.33 A large smegma cyst at the dorsum of the penis.

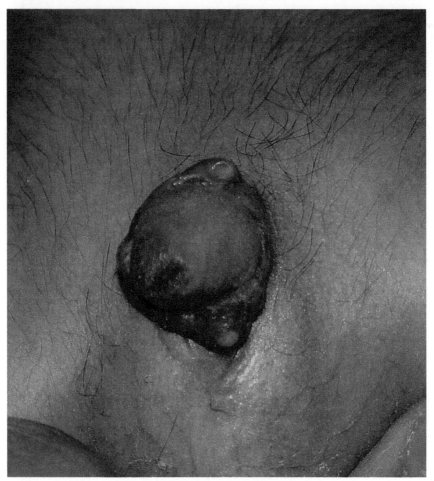

FIG. 10.34 Multiple small smegma cysts.

POST-CIRCUMCISION PENILE LYMPHOEDEMA

Generally, lymphoedema of the external genitalia is an unusual problem in countries where endemic filariasis is rarely experienced. The abnormal retention of lymphatic fluid in subcutaneous tissue as a result of lymphatic obstruction can cause swelling, pain, disfigurement, difficulties in urination and later on a decrease in potency. Lymphoedema may be idiopathic or secondary to inflammation, surgical incision, neoplasm, radiation, hypoproteinemia, venous thrombosis and other medical conditions.

Preputial cutting severs the lymph vessels of the penile skin, and it may interrupt the circulation of lymph and sometimes cause different grades of penile lymphoedema,[24] which is a painful, disfiguring condition in which the remaining skin of the penis swells with trapped lymph fluid. A few cases had been reported in the literature complicating MC, but we diagnosed a few cases with a variable extension and different forms of presentations (Fig. 10.36).

On the other hand, cutaneous lymphangiectasia (CL) or acquired lymphangioma is another lymphatic malformation, mostly congenital, whereas acquired CL occurs because of the obstruction of deeper lymphatic vessels secondary to other causes.[25] It is characterized by the presence of a circumscribed eruption of thin-walled, translucent vesicles and ranges from clear, fluid-filled blisters to smooth, flesh-coloured nodules, sometimes with a coexisting lymphoedema. Mostly, CL is asymptomatic but pruritus, burning or painful lesion and sometimes a foul-smelling viscous discharge may also occur. We have only one case diagnosed as

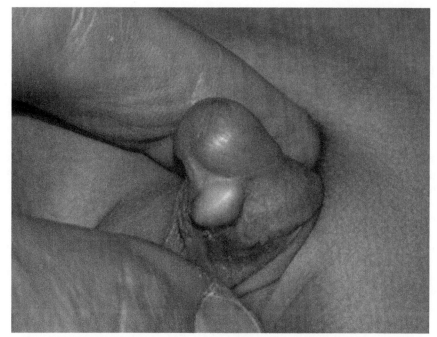

FIG. 10.35 Post-circumcision smegma cyst in the ventral penile surface looks like a mucoid penile cyst.

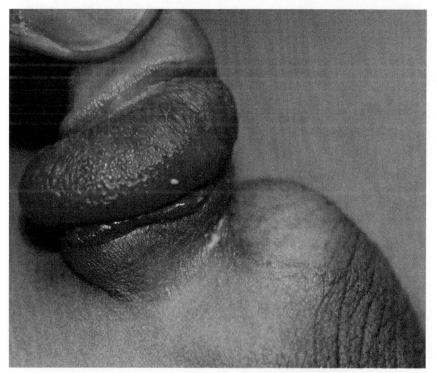

FIG. 10.36 A localized lymphoedema of excess inner prepuce after guillotine male circumcision.

having CL in a previously normal adolescent, who was circumcised at the age of 10 years under general anaesthesia and developed CL at the scar of circumcision 2 months after the procedure, with progressive extension of the characteristic skin lesions in the penile and scrotal skin, which resulted in an ugly scar at the coronal sulcus; histopathologic findings confirmed the diagnosis of CL (Fig. 10.37).

Pathophysiology

There are two lymphatic systems in the penis: the superficial system and the deep system. The superficial system drains the prepuce and the skin of the penis, and it flows into the superomedial zone of the superficial inguinal nodes. The deep system drains the glans, runs beneath the deep fascia and flows both directly into the pelvic nodes and the superficial inguinal nodes. These anatomic structures can explain the discrepancy between the severely involved penile skin and the intact glans, as observed in Fig. 10.38, where the extensive excision of penile skin during MC results in lymphoedema of the remnant penile and scrotal skin, while the glans is minimally affected (Fig. 10.38).

The lymphatic vessels of the superficial dermal plexus drain a fixed area of skin through the vertical collecting lymphatics to the deep plexus. The damage to deep lymphatic vessels leads to back pressure and dermal backflow, with subsequent dilatation of the upper dermal lymphatics. Because circumferential excision of the penile skin above the deep fascia does not interfere with the deep lymphatic system, secondary penile lymphoedema is unusual.[26]

Diagnosis

The diagnosis is mainly clinical aided by the histopathologic finding of dilated lymphatics in the dermis during surgical treatment.

Post-MC lymphoedema could be classified according to its extension into

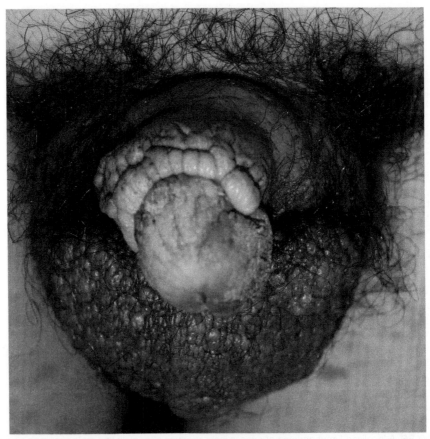

FIG. 10.37 A case of cutaneous lymphangiectasia complicating adult male circumcision, with the main brunt of the lesion at the circumcision scar and with an extension to the scrotal skin.

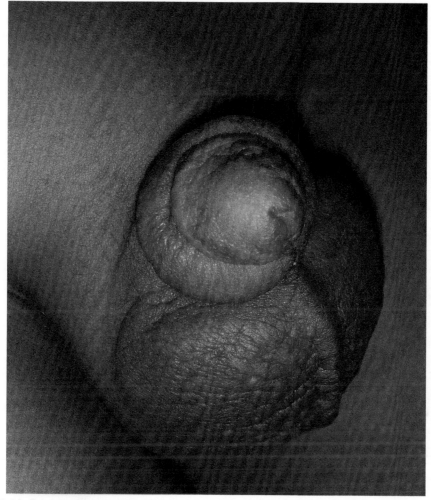

FIG. 10.38 Extensive excision of the outer prepuce and penile skin results in secondary lymphoedema of the scrotum, with minimal glandular involvement.

- lymphoedema of the excess remnant prepuce (Fig. 10.36),
- penile lymphoedema,
- penoscrotal lymphoedema (Figs. 10.38 and 10.39),
- CL (Fig. 10.37).

Differential Diagnosis

Lymphoedema detected after MC should be differentiated from cases of congenital primary lymphoedema (lymphoedema praecox), which is a rare anomaly and may be present since birth or may develop later but unrecognized before performing MC and only manifested or could be aggravated after the surgical trauma of MC, as circumcision may have initiated and accelerated the lymphatic obstruction leading to oedema[27] (Fig. 10.39).

Post-MC lymphoedema should also be differentiated from cases of angioneurotic oedema, which may accidentally follow MC due to local or systemic causes, such as insect bites or drug eruption, in the latter case, the condition usually affects other organs with itching and responding early to antihistaminic medications[28] (Fig. 10.40).

Lymphangiectasia has to be differentiated from herpes genitalis, genital warts and molluscum contagiosum.

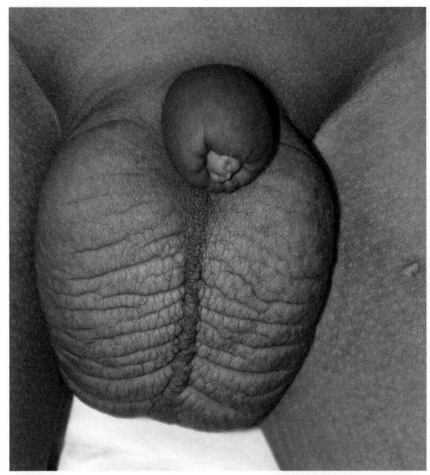

FIG. 10.39 A circumcised child with congenital primary lymphoedema affecting the penile and scrotal skin.

Treatment

Regardless of the cause, lymphoedema is not fatal, but its chronic nature makes the patient miserable. Treatment should be directed towards the cause and aimed for reduction of the underlying oedema and control of infection.

Management of isolated penile lymphoedema is challenging, and medical treatments include the use of oral antibiotics for identified infectious pathogens, empirical antibiotics for presumed subacute genital infections, oral steroids and topical steroid application limited to areas with cutaneous lesions.[29] Although various methods of lymphangioplasty have been described by several authors, they are technically difficult and unreliable and are therefore not often performed. The most common approach is excision of all the involved skin and subcutaneous tissue to the level of Buck fascia followed by coverage of the genitalia with local tissue flaps or skin grafts.[30]

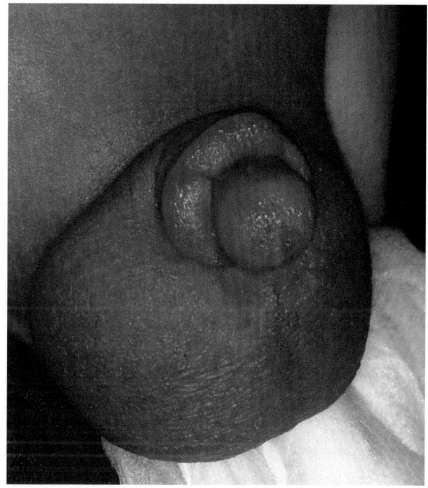

FIG. 10.40 A case of post-male circumcision angioneurotic oedema affecting the preputial remnant and extending to the penile and scrotal skin, which resolved after conservative measures.

REFERENCES

1. Ulman İ, Ali T. How do I get a perfect cosmetic result after circumcision? In: Rané A, et al., eds. *Practical Tips in Urology*. London: Springer-Verlag; 2017. https://doi.org/10.1007/978-1-4471-4348-2_15.

2. Fergusson DM, Lawton JM, Shannon FT. Neonatal circumcision and penile problems: an 8-year longitudinal study. *Pediatrics*. 1988;81:537−541.

3. Akyol I, Soydan H, Kocoglu H, Ates F, Karademir K, Baykal K. A novel tool to predict the cosmetic outcome after circumcision: penile visibility index. *Int J Clin Med*. 2014;5:605−610. https://doi.org/10.4236/ijcm.2014.510082.

4. Pieretti RV, Goldstein AM, Pieretti-Vanmarcke R. Late complications of newborn circumcision: a common and avoidable problem. *Pediatr Surg Int*. 2010;26(5):515−518.

5. Krill AJ, Palmer LS, Palmer JS. Complications of circumcision. *Sci World J*. 2011;11:11. https://doi.org/10.1100/2011/373829. Article ID 373829.

6. Draaijers LJ, Tempelman FR, Botman YA, et al. The patient and observer scar assessment scale: a reliable and feasible tool for scar evaluation. *Plast Reconstr Surg*. 2004;113(7):1960−1965.

7. Maizels M, Zaontz M, Donovan J. Surgical correction of the buried penis: description of a classification system and a technique to correct the disorder. *J Urol*. 1986;136:268−271.

8. Williams CP, Richardson BG, Bukowski TP. Importance of identifying the inconspicuous penis: prevention of circumcision complications. *Urology*. 2000;56:140−143. https://doi.org/10.1016/S0090-4295(00)00601-4.

9. Borsellino A, Spagnoli A, Vallasciani S, Martini L, Ferro F. Surgical approach to concealed penis: technical refinements

and outcome. *Urology.* 2007;69:1195−1198. https://doi.org/10.1016/j.urology.2007.01.065.

10. Van Howe RS. Variability in penile appearance and penile findings: a prospective study. *Br J Urol.* 1997;80:776−782.

11. Blalock HJ, et al. Outpatient management of phimosis following newborn circumcision. *J Urol.* 169(6): 2332 − 2334.

12. Skrodzka M, et al. How to do a circumcision, when the foreskin is welded to the glans. *J Sexual Med.* 15(7): S179 − S180.

13. Bragg BN, Leslie SW. *Paraphimosis NCBI Bookshelf. A Service of the National Library of Medicine, National Institutes of Health. StatPearls [Internet].* Treasure Island (FL): StatPearls Publishing; June 2017. Bookshelf ID: NBK459233 PMID: 29083645.

14. Talini C, Antunes LA, de Carvalho BCN, et al. Circumcision: postoperative complications that required reoperation. *Einstein.* 2018;16(3):eAO4241. https://doi.org/10.1590/S1679-45082018AO4241.

15. Palmisano F, Gadda F, Spinelli MG, Montanari E. Glans penis necrosis following paraphimosis: a rare case with brief literature review. *Urol Case Rep.* 2018;16:57−58. https://doi.org/10.1016/j.eucr.2017.09.016.

16. Hayashi Y, Kojima Y, Mizuno K, Kohri K. Prepuce: phimosis, paraphimosis, and circumcision. *Scientific World J.* 2011;11:289−301. https://doi.org/10.1100/tsw.2011.31.

17. Warwick DJ, Dickson WA. Keloid of the penis after circumcision. *Postgrad Med.* 1993;69(809):236−237.

18. Yong M, Afshar K, MacNeily A, Arneja JS. Management of pediatric penile keloid. *Can Urol Assoc J.* 2013;7(9−10): E618−E620. https://doi.org/10.5489/cuaj.408.

19. Hypertrophic scar and keloid formation after male circumcision - a case report. *Eur J Plast Surg.* 2009; 32(4):213−215. https://doi.org/10.1007/s00238-008-0319-y.

20. Wright J. How smegma serves the penis. *Sexology.* 1970;37: 50−53.

21. Aridogan IA, Ilkit M, Izol V, Ates A, Demirhindi H. Glans penis and prepuce colonisation of yeast fungi in a paediatric population: pre- and post circumcision results. *Mycoses.* 2009;52(1):49−52.

22. Baky FMA. The spectrum of genital median raphe anomalies among infants undergoing ritual circumcision. *J Pediatr Urol.* 2013;9:e872−e877. https://doi.org/10.1016/j.jpurol.2012.11.018.

23. Fahmy M: Smegma in Congenital Anomalies of the Penis, Illustrative Textbook. Springer International Publishing, Pages 237−240. ISBN 978-3-319-43310-3

24. Shulman J, Ben-Hur N, Neuman Z. Surgical complications of circumcision. *Am J Dis Child.* 1964;107:149−154. https://doi.org/10.1001/archpedi 1964.02080060151007.

25. Arya S, Nyati A, Moti, Lal B. Cutaneous lymphangiectasia of genitalia: a rare occurrence. *J Assoc Phys India.* 2018; (66):94.

26. Dewire D, Lepor H. Anatomic considerations of the penis and its lymphatic drainage. *Urol Clin.* 1992;19:211−219.

27. Serkan Y, Gaye T, Tayfun A. Circumcision as an unusual cause of penile lymphedema. *Ann Plast Surg.* 2003;50(6): 665−666. Letters.

28. Fahmy M. Penile lymphedema. In: *Congenital Anomalies of the Penis.* Cham: Springer; 2017. https://doi.org/10.1007/978-3-319-43310-3_18.

29. Garaffa G, Christopher N, Ralph DJ. The management of genital lymphoedema. *BJU Int.* 2008;102:480−484. https://doi.org/10.1111/j.1464-410X.2008.07559.x.

30. Modolin M, Mitre AI, da Silva JC, et al. Surgical treatment of lymphedema of the penis and scrotum. *Clinics.* 2006;61: 289−294.

CHAPTER 11

Circumcision Scars and Aesthetic Concerns

JONATHAN A. ALLAN, PhD

ABSTRACT

In North America, it is fairly common to imagine the uncircumcised, or the intact, penis as 'ugly'. Numerous examples can be found in popular cultures that refer to the uncircumcised penis and its foreskin as abject, disgusting, dirty, etc. As such, the circumcised penis has become something of a norm in North America, especially the United States where in the words of one scholar, 'circumcision is consistent with American notions of good parenting'. Likewise, the foreskin has seemingly disappeared form medical textbooks, as noted by J.R. Taylor, A.P. Lockwood and A.J. Taylor: 'The current tendency to eliminate the prepuce from anatomy textbooks reflects the popular emphasis on the glans; perhaps the wrinkling and pleating of the retracted prepuce, like unwanted hair, is an affront to good taste or simply superfluous to requirements.' What all this assumes, of course, is that the circumcised men are aesthetically superior and that all circumcisions will necessarily result in this aesthetic improvement — in this logic, then, there are never any mistakes or accidents. However, as has been well documented, circumcision complications do arise, and sometimes they leave the penis with scars, which can become an aesthetic concern; indeed, the correction, as it were, can become a new problem. This chapter thus considers the (possible) ugliness of the circumcised penis.

KEYWORDS

Aesthetics; Circumcision; Foreskin; Scars.

In North America, it is fairly common to imagine that the uncircumcised penis is 'ugly'.[1] Numerous examples can be found in popular cultures that refer to the uncircumcised penis and its foreskin as abject, disgusting and dirty. As such, the circumcised penis has become something of a norm in North America, especially in the United States where 'circumcision is consistent with

the American notions of good parenting'.[2] Indeed, as noted by J.R. Taylor, A.P. Lockwood and A.J. Taylor, the foreskin has disappeared from medical textbooks:

> The current tendency to eliminate the prepuce from anatomy textbooks reflects the popular emphasis on the glans; perhaps the wrinkling and pleating of the retracted prepuce, like unwanted hair, is an affront to good taste or simply superfluous to requirements.[3]

What all this assumes, of course, is that the circumcised penis is aesthetically superior and that all circumcisions will necessarily result in this same aesthetic improvement — in this logic, then, there are never any mistakes or accidents. However, as has been well-documented, circumcision complications do arise, and sometimes they leave the penis with scars, which can become an aesthetic concern; indeed, the correction, as it were, can become a new problem. This chapter thus considers the ugliness of the circumcised penis, especially when complications arise.

A NOTE ON TERMINOLOGY

I use the term 'uncircumcised' to refer to the penis that has not been circumcised. I recognize, however, that this terminology is problematic for some, especially those in the anti-circumcision community. Wallace[4] has proposed that we ought to use three distinct terms to refer to different types of penises: 'intact (those in the natural state), circumcised (those with the prepuce removed), and uncircumcised (those with a restored prepuce or pseudo-prepuce).' I recognize that for Wallace these distinctions are important, and he is not alone. In one article published in the Australian Forum, a man explains, 'I really resent the calling of a man who has a natural penis with foreskin … 'uncircumcised' as if it was something that had to be done!'[5] Likewise, Lander[6] explains that using the term 'uncircumcised' is 'irrational' because it requires that one 'define the normal as "not operated upon"' and thus argues that 'the normal male should be addressed as such, or referred to as

Complications in Male Circumcision. https://doi.org/10.1016/B978-0-323-68127-8.00011-9

"intact"'. However, it seems to me that 'uncircumcised' is the commonly accepted terminology for a penis that has retained its foreskin, even if there are a growing number of men who would prefer a term such as 'intact' or 'natural'. Moreover, what is missing from Wallace's typologies is the case of *apposthia*, in which, the neonate is born without a foreskin. Regardless, what should be clear is that the profession should respect the term or terms that an individual uses for himself.

A NOTE ON APPROACH

This article is established in the social sciences and humanities, rather than the medical sciences; however, I believe it contributes to both disburses and fields of inquiry and practice. Just as I have done in my research on the uncircumcised penis, I draw on a range of sources that may be unfamiliar to those trained in the medical sciences, or even sources that might never be quoted in the medical sciences, for any number of reasons. As a scholar, I am as likely to work with an ethnographic study as I am to work with a sex advice column in a popular magazine. I think it is important that wherever we come from that we are engaging with a wide range of materials because we likely will encounter a wide range of perspectives in the people we engage with, the audiences with whom we speak and the patients who are cared for by the medical profession.

CIRCUMCISION

Circumcision is perhaps the world's first surgery, and most would likely agree that it is, at the very least, probably one of the oldest of all surgical procedures.[7] Incidentally, decircumcision, or foreskin restoration, is likely the oldest, and thus, the first aesthetic surgery as Gilman has argued.[8] Hutson[9] notes, 'circumcision has a long history in ancient societies of the Middle East, and is likely to have arisen as an early public health measure for preventing recurrent balanitis, caused by sand accumulating under the foreskin.' Of course, circumcision has also been 'a major part of the ritual for such religions as Judaism, Christianity and Islam', and as Hutson noted, 'it is probably not accident that all of these arose in the Middle East.'[9] Today, circumcision is carried out not only for religious reasons but also, and importantly, for secular reasons, such as 'the father's desire for the baby to look like himself'[9] which is one of the most common reasons, as well as a fear of the locker room, wherein a boy would have a penis that looks different from that of those around him. For example, a 1987 article found that the most popular reason (46%) for circumcision 'was wanting our son to resemble other males'.[10] Likewise, a 2014 study

published in the Pediatric Surgery International found that little has changed. In this study, we learn that the most common reasons for circumcision were 'to be like dad' (69%) and social acceptance among peers (69%), and the other reasons included health and in only 11% of cases were religious reasons given for routine neonatal circumcision in the hospital setting.[11] Indeed, in a 2015 study published in The Journal of Perinatal Education, the reasons for circumcision remain similar: '[P]arents choose circumcision for their newborn sons for the child to have the same appearance as his father, to reduce his risk for infection, and because of beliefs about hygiene.'[12] At bottom, then, it must be admitted that 'a man's perception of his genitalia has a significant effect on self-esteem and sexual identity',[13] which is why it is important that clinicians consider the question of aesthetics with regard to circumcision decisions.

CIRCUMCISION RISKS AND AESTHETIC CONSIDERATIONS

Given that 'circumcision is the most frequently performed operation in the world',[14] in addition to the influence on 'self-esteem and sexual identity',[13] it seems valuable and important to consider the impact of the operation. From the outset, it should be recalled that the overall complication rate of 1.5% is low; however, as Schröder notes, "given the number of circumcisions performed worldwide, the number of affected children is enormous."

In a survey completed by the National Organization to Halt the Abuse and Routine Mutilation of Males, respondents reported wide-ranging physical consequences from their circumcisions. Among the most significant consequences were prominent scarring (33%), insufficient penile skin for a comfortable erection (27%), erectile curvature from uneven skin loss (16%), pain and bleeding upon erection/manipulation (17%), painful skin bridges (12%) and others, e.g. bevelling deformities of the glans, meatal stenosis and recurrent nonspecific urethritis (20%).[15]

Admittedly, this data is likely biased insofar as the study was conducted by an organization that has the explicit mandate of putting an end to routine neonatal circumcision. But what is valuable in this list is a series of reasons, commonly presented, against circumcision. Then the risks of circumcision are prominent scarring, insufficient penile skin for a comfortable erection and erectile curvature. Some of these reasons are more physical than aesthetic, but it is difficult to distinguish between the two, especially for a man in whom his penis has provided challenges to his self-esteem and sexual identity.[13]

When we think about circumcision complications, we ought to move beyond the merely functional 'does the penis still work?' and towards other adjacent or orthogonal considerations, for instance, aesthetics. I argue, it would be advantageous to begin to think through the aesthetics of circumcision, especially given how frequent the reasons for circumcision are, in one sense or another, aesthetic, for instance, the circumcised penis looks better than the uncircumcised penis or for a son to look like his father and/or brothers. Although the latter reason may speak to community, it is also an aesthetic argument, which is to say, about appearances.

SCARS

Circumcisions, as we likely know, are not uniform; that is, not all circumcised penises look the same, even though they will look similar. There are different methods for circumcision, which will produce different results, at least aesthetically speaking. Gérard Zwang, for instance, notes that 'the scar created by ritual circumcision, practiced in a workmanlike manner by non-doctors—be they mohels or barbers—is usually unsightly, torturous, and irregular, especially if it has suppurated.'[16] Zwang's concern is ritual circumcision, but many of these same thoughts appear in critiques of medical circumcision. Nonetheless, what remains true is that circumcision does affect the aesthetics of the penis – even arguments for circumcision are often about improving upon the apparent ugliness of the un-circumcised penis.

In the cases of medical circumcisions, there are a few methods that have become commonplace, namely, the Mogen clamp, the Gomco clamp and the Plastibell, as well as less common modes such as the Sheldon clamp, which produces a guillotine-type circumcision.[17] Given these different tools, it stands to reason that

circumcision will not be uniform. Likewise, it has been observed that although the 'many techniques of circumcision have a common goal: to remove equal amounts of inner and outer epithelial preputial tissue in a rapid, minimally traumatic and haemostatic fashion', it must be admitted that there is a 'fairly high [complication] rate (1.5 to 15%), [which] reflects the fact that the procedure is often performed by an inexperienced individual without attention to basic surgical principles.'[17] Incidentally, the Canadian newspaper, The Globe and Mail, reported that 'few, if any, jurisdiction in Canada require physicians to undergo formal training before performing circumcision.'[18]

Needless to say, given these dynamics, it is not surprising that circumcision results vary and complications do happen. The circumcision scar may appear in different places along the penis; for instance, one survey noted that one respondent had the scar close behind the glans, whereas the other's scar was 25 mm back from it (Fig. 11.1).[19]

Additionally, although it is true that 'the Gomco clamp and the Plastibell devices produce an even circular cut', it must also be acknowledged that 'if applied crookedly can result in cosmetic problems.'[20] Research has shown that the Gomco clamp has an overall complication rate of 1.9% and that the Plastibell's overall complication rate range from 2.4% to 5%.[21] In what follows, I focus on a few of these cosmetic problems, specifically missing frenulum, skin bridges or adhesions, two-toned and pigmentation variation and damage to the glans penis.

Missing Frenulum

A *frenulum* is 'a small fold of integument or mucous membrane that limits the move of an organ or part', and in the case of the penis, 'the frenulum tethers the

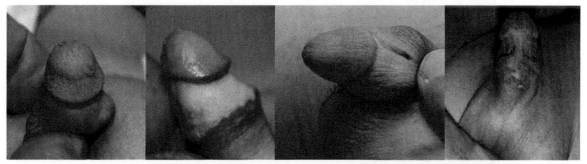

FIG. 11.1 Sequence of post circumcision scars from distal to proximal. From right to left: a scared glans penis, scarring of the excess inner prepuce, a visible stitch sinus in excess prepuce, and distal scaring in the penile shaft. (Photo credit: Mohamed Fahmy.)

foreskin and brings it back into position following retraction. The frenulum is continuous with the ridged band, which is a highly innervated pleated tissue just inside the opening of the foreskin. The frenulum and ridged band may have the highest concentration of fine-touch and other specialized neuroreceptors in the male body.'[22] (Figs. 11.2 and 11.3).

As such, the frenulum is often described as the king of all sensitive areas[23] or as the so-called 'G-spot' of males,[24] which is why it so often appears in sex advice columns in magazines and sex manuals. More specifically, 'the frenulum is, by design, a little on the short side, so that during an erection and the swelling of the glans there is a pull on the band.'[23] Although not

necessarily an aesthetic concern, for many, it is most certainly a sexual and erotic concern.

Importantly, the frenulum is not removed during all circumcisions, as O'Hara and O'Hara note, 'the tip of the foreskin, and *some or all of the frenulum*, are routinely removed as part of circumcision.'[25] Likewise, Hammond and Carmack note that 'the highly erogenous frenulum, often preserved in adult circumcision, is frequently ablated in neonatal circumcision due to the smaller size of the undeveloped penis.'[26] Neonatal circumcision, thus, presents an interesting aspect to the ongoing debates about circumcision. It would seem that more care is taken with the adult penis, if we accept the claims of Hammond and Carmack, which

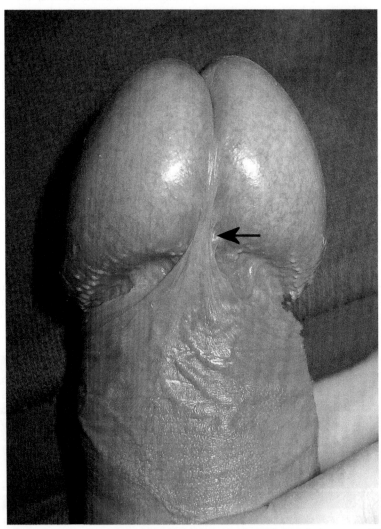

FIG. 11.2 Intact frenulum. (Source: https://upload.wikimedia.org/wikipedia/commons/5/54/Image_of_frenulum.jpg)

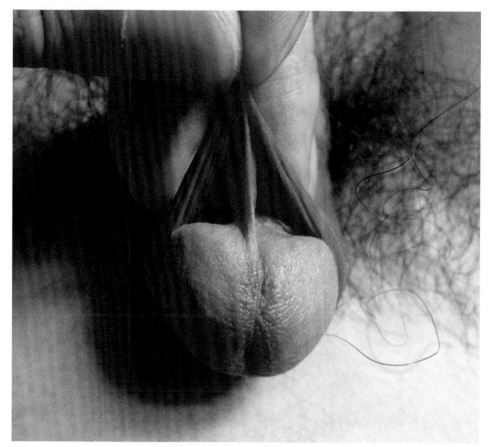

FIG. 11.3 Stretched frenulum with intact prepuce. (Source: https://upload.wikimedia.org/wikipedia/commons/0/02/BPXD_dicksoft_stress.JPG)

undoubtedly has an effect and influence on self-esteem, aesthetics and sexuality.

Skin Bridges

Ponsky and colleagues[27,28] noted, 'penile adhesions are common after circumcision' and found that 28% of the boys they evaluated had some kind of penile adhesion, including skin bridges. Of the '254 boys 25 were referred for evaluation of penile adhesions, skin bridges, or other circumcision related issues.'[28] Gerharz and Haarman[29] note that one 'adverse result of circumcision is the formation of cutaneous bridges between the glans penis and the penile shaft' and explain that 'prominent skin bridges are aesthetically disturbing and may lead to tethering of the erect penis, with pain or penile curvature.'

In Fig. 11.4, the skin bridge is relatively minor and is mostly visible because of the erect state. However, the skin bridge may create discomfort to and/or curvature of the penis. The skin bridge thus shows a deviation from the norm of a circumcised penis or an ideal circumcised penis. Romberg[30] explains that a skin bridge 'is a complication in healing of the wound, by which a piece of skin from the shaft of the penis has become attached to the glans, or another point along the shaft, forming a "bridge" that must be surgically corrected.'

Two-Toned and Pigmentation Variations

One additional aesthetic concern, for some men, is what might be understood as a 'two-toned' penis, wherein the penis has two distinct colours, often divided by the circumcision scar (Figs. 11.5–11.7).

This two-toned penis may not be an ideal one, and it may be considered an ugly or aesthetic concern for some men. In a survey completed by National

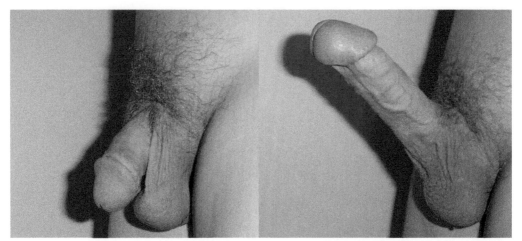

FIG. 11.4 Post circumcision small skin bridge, visible in erect penis. (Source: https://upload.wikimedia.org/wikipedia/commons/4/4b/Flaccid-erect.jpg)

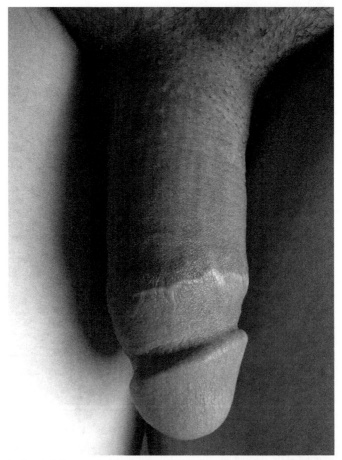

FIG. 11.5 Toned pigmentation and visible scar in flacid penis. (Source: https://upload.wikimedia.org/wikipedia/commons/0/06/Circumcised_flaccid.jpg)

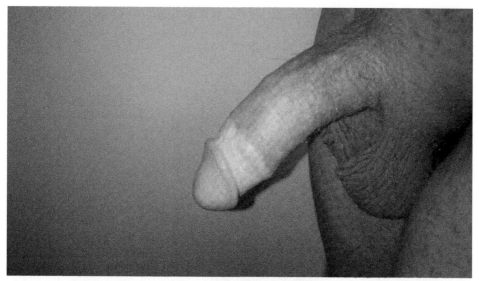

FIG. 11.6 Toned pigmentation and visible scar on erected penis. (Source: https://commons.wikimedia.org/wiki/Category:Circumcised_human_penis#/media/File:Circumcised_Penis_2.jpg)

Organization of Restoring Men, UK, 74% of the respondents were dissatisfied with the appearance of their circumcised penises, and particularly, 26% complained about the variation in skin colour.[31] In the cases shown in Figs. 11.5–11.7, the penis is clearly functional; indeed, in Fig. 11.7, an erect penis is presented (with the frenulum intact). In each case, the circumcision scar is clearly visible. This scar, although likely not of concern for many, is certainly a concern for some; one respondent in a survey explained, 'the physical scar is hideous, but the emotional scar equates to rape'.[32] We should not be quick to dismiss these attitudes or ideas because for these men, they are genuinely held beliefs.

The Glans

Perhaps one of the most extreme examples of scarring and aesthetic concerns would be the example of the amputation of the glans penis, which is recognized as a rare circumcision complication.[33] One case study notes that 'the Sheldon clamp was placed over the prepuce, and the foreskin was pulled through the clamp and crushed. A scalpel was used to excise the prepuce. It was immediately recognized that the distal third of the penile glans had been surgically amputated.'[17] Another study notes a similar result in six cases that used the Mogen clamp. The Sheldon and Mogen clamps, unlike the Plastibell or the Gomco clamp, do not have a glans protective mechanism that minimizes its inclusion and injury during circumcision.[34]

In their work, Salle and colleagues observed that Glans amputation during neonatal circumcision is a potentially devastating complication that appears to be particularly associated with the use of the Mogen clamp. They proposed that glans amputation can be prevented by careful preparation of the foreskin with complete lysis of ventral preputial adhesions before the placement of the clamp in order to avoid traction and inadvertent entrapment.[35]

To be certain, complications do not arise with the Mogen or Sheldon clamp alone. One case study speaks of a child (4 years) who 'had had a Plastibell circumcision 10 days previously' and that 'he had rested his penis on the toilet bowl, when a large wooden seat fell on the glans where the Plastibell ring was. This resulted in traumatic amputation of the glans.'[36] In such cases, then, undoubtedly, aesthetic considerations will remain and will need to be attended to. There will be scars from the reattachment of the glans (if possible), or there will be a noticeable absence of a part of the glans.

CONCLUSION: AESTHETICS MATTER

While the measure of a good circumcision might well be functionality, it is important that we take into account the aesthetic concerns. Brennan[37] notes that 'getting "botched" is a persistent anxiety of our augmentation-by-surgery age', and although the incidence of circumcision complications is minimal, it is not insignificant,

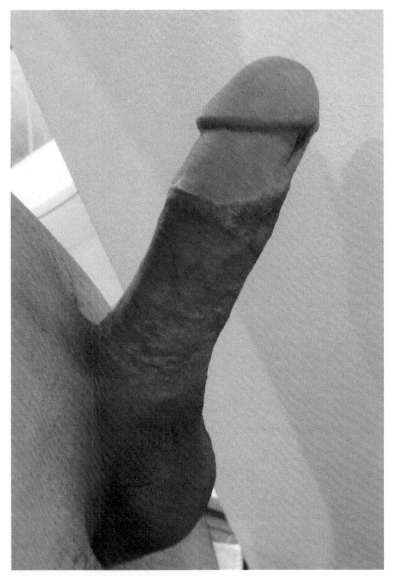

FIG. 11.7 Prominent color change on circumcised penis, with two circumcision scars following a second circumcision to correct inadequate foreskin removed after initial circumcision. The frenulum has been trimmed but retained. (Source: https://commons.wikimedia.org/wiki/Category:Circumcised_human_penis#/media/File:Circumcisedtwice.jpg)

especially with regard to self-esteem and sexual identity,[13] as well as the perspectives and ideas of others, which, of course, have an influence on self-esteem. There is, of course, a significant body of scholarship that has noted, 'thoughts about one's body, including thoughts specific to one's own genitals, have been linked to men's sexual function.'[38] Unsurprisingly, then, 'the role of body image in men's sexual lives extends also to their penis specifically'; however, 'genital body image has typically focussed on appearance of the penis or penis length.'[38] Indeed, as Bossio and Pukall[38] note, 'little research has empirically explored the potential role of circumcision status in a man's body appraisal of his body image, particularly as body image relates to sexual functioning.' I certainly agree with Bossio and Pukall, but as this chapter has sought to demonstrate that not all circumcisions are the same, we need to focus not only on circumcision but also on the quality of circumcision, which includes taking into account aesthetic or cosmetic matters, as well as sexual and functional concerns. As such, circumcision complications should not be treated lightly, even if the penis is functional. We might do well to think about the adjacent concerns: aesthetics, sexuality and self-esteem.

ACKNOWLEDGMENT

This research was undertaken, in part, thanks to funding from the Canada Research Chairs program.

REFERENCES

1. Allan, JA. The foreskin aesthetic, or ugliness reconsidered. *Men Masculinities.* Online First: http://journals.sagepub.com/doi/full/10.1177/1097184X17753038.
2. Waldeck SE. Social norm theory and male circumcision: why parents circumcise. *Am J Bioeth.* 2003;3(2):57.
3. Taylor JR, Lockwood AP, Taylor AJ. The prepuce: specialized mucosa of the penis and its loss to circumcision. *Br J Urol.* 1996;77:294.
4. Wallace WG. An undeniable need for change: the case for redefining human penis types: intact, circumcised, and uncircumcised (all three forms exists and all are different). *Clin Anat.* 2015;28:564.
5. James B. Circumcision—what you think. *Australian Forum.* 1989;2(11):12.
6. Lander MM. The human prepuce. In: Denniston GC, Milos MF, eds. *Sexual Mutilations: A Human Tragedy.* New York: Plenum Press; 1997:77.
7. Gerharz EW, Haarman C. The first cut is the deepest? Medicolegal aspects of male circumcision. *BJU Int.* 2000;86:332.
8. Gilman SL. Decircumcision: the first aesthetic surgery. *Mod Jud.* 1997;17(3):201–210.
9. Hutson JM. Circumcision: a surgeon's perspective. *J Med Ethics.* 2004;30:238.
10. Brodbarnemzer J, Conrad P, Tenenbaum S. American circumcision practices and social reality. *Sociol Soc Res.* 1987;71(4):276.
11. Freeman JJ, et al. Newborn circumcision outcomes: are parents satisfied with the results? *Pediatr Surg Int.* 2014; 30(3):334.
12. Mitchell TM, Beal C. Shared decision making for routine infant circumcision: a pilot study. *J Perinat Educ.* 2015; 24(3):189.
13. Alter GJ, Salgado CJ, Chim H. Aesthetic surgery of the male genitalia. *Semin Plast Surg.* 2011;25(3):189 (Thieme Medical Publishers).
14. Schröder A. Circumcision: case against surgery without medical indication. In: Bolnick DA, et al., eds. *Surgical Guide to Circumcision.* London: Springer-Verlag; 2012:188.
15. Hammond T. A preliminary poll of men circumcised in infancy or childhood. *BJU Int.* 1999;83(suppl. 1):86.
16. Zwang G. Function and erotic consequences of sexual mutilations. In: Denniston GC, Milos MF, eds. *Sexual Mutilations: A Human Tragedy.* New York: Plenum Press; 1997:74.
17. Gluckman GR, et al. Newborn penile glans amputation during circumcision and successful reattachment. *J Urol.* 1995;153:778.
18. Weeks C. *Canadian Doctors Need More Formal Training in Circumcision.* The Globe and Mail; September 21, 2015. Online: https://www.theglobeandmail.com/life/health-and-fitness/health/canadian-doctors-need-more-formal-training-in-circumcision/article26454085/.
19. James B. Circumcision—what you think. *Australian Forum.* 1989;2(11):13.
20. Romberg R. *Circumcision: The Painful Dilemma.* South Hadley, MA: Bergin and Garvey Publishers; 1985:228.
21. Freedman, Lerman, and Bergman. 47–48.
22. Van Howe RS. Frenulum. In: Kimmel M, Milrod C, Kennedy A, eds. *The Cultural Encyclopedia of the Penis.* Lanham: Rowman & Littlefield; 2014:75.
23. Gralla O. *Happy Down Below: Everything You Want to Know About the Penis and Other Bits, Trans. Jamie McIntosh.* Vancouver: Greystone Books; 2018:39.
24. McGrath K. The frenular delta: a new preputial structure. In: Denniston GC, Hodges FM, Milos MF, eds. *Understanding Circumcision: A Multi-Disciplinary Approach to a Multi-Dimensional Problem.* New York: Kluwer Academic/Plenum Publishers; 2001:205.
25. O'Hara K, O'Hara J. The effect of male circumcision on the sexual enjoyment of the female partner. *BJU Int.* 1999; 83(suppl. 1):80.
26. Hammond T, Carmack A. Long-term adverse outcomes from neonatal circumcision reported in a survey of 1,008 men: an overview of health and human rights implications. *Int J Hum Right.* 2017;21(2):194.
27. Ponsky LE, Ross JH, Knipper N, Kay R. Penile adhesions after neonatal circumcision. *J Urol.* 2000;164:495.
28. Ponsky LE, Ross JH, Knipper N, Kay R. Penile adhesions after neonatal circumcision. *J Urol.* 2000;164:496.
29. Gerharz EW, Haarman C. The first cut is the deepest? Medicolegal aspects of male circumcision. *BJU Int.* 2000;86:336–337.
30. Romberg R. *Circumcision: The Painful Dilemma.* South Hadley, MA: Bergin and Garvey Publishers; 1985:221.
31. Warren JP. NORM UK and the medical case against circumcision. In: Denniston GC, Milos MF, eds. *Sexual Mutilations: A Human Tragedy.* New York: Plenum Press; 1997:95.
32. Hammond T, Carmack A. Long-term adverse outcomes from neonatal circumcision reported in a survey of 1,008 men: an overview of health and human rights implications. *Int J Hum Right.* 2017;21(2):200.
33. Faydaci G, et al. Amputation of glans penis: a rare circumcision complication and successful management with

primary anastomosis and hyperbaric oxygen therapy. *Korean J Urol.* 2011;52(2):147.

34. Joao L, Salle P, et al. Glans amputation during routine neonatal circumcision: mechanism of injury and strategy for prevention. *J Pediatr Urol.* 2013;9:765.
35. Joao L, Salle P, et al. Glans amputation during routine neonatal circumcision: mechanism of injury and strategy for prevention. *J Pediatr Urol.* 2013;9:767.
36. Paul C, et al. Surgical repair of traumatic amputation of the glans. *Urology.* 2011;77(6):1472.
37. Brennan J. Porn penis, malformed penis. *Porn Studies.* 2017:6. Online First.
38. Bossio JA, Pukall CF. Attitude toward one's circumcision status is more important than actual circumcision status for men's body image and sexual function. *Arch Sex Behav.* 2018;47:772.

CHAPTER 12

Post-Male Circumcision Penile Injuries

MOHAMED A BAKY FAHMY, MD, FRCS

ABSTRACT

Penile injuries after circumcision are usually disastrous, resulting in a sort of disability, and are mainly iatrogenic, discovered during or immediately after the procedure, if a post circumcision dressing applied too tightly to a contaminated and infected wound and left on for too long, it can lead to compression of the urethra resulting in skin necrosis and urethral ischaemia. Penile injury complications are usually combined lesions affecting more than one entity and are commonly reported in neonatal male circumcision, especially in those performed by nonmedical staff. However, there are many cases of severe injuries and even penile destructions caused by medical personnel in highly qualified centers.

KEYWORDS

Ablatio penis; Corporal injury; Fournier gangrene; Glans injury; Iatrogenic hypospadias; Meatal injury; Penile amputation; Penile skin loss; Urethral injuries; Vascular injuries and ischaemia.

Penile injuries after circumcision are usually disastrous, resulting in a sort of disability, and are mainly iatrogenic, discovered during or immediately after the procedure, if a post circumcision dressing applied too tightly to a contaminated and infected wound and left on for too long, it can lead to compression of the urethra resulting in skin necrosis and urethral ischaemia. Penile injury complications are usually combined lesions affecting more than one entity and are commonly reported with neonatal male circumcision (MC), especially in those performed by nonmedical staff. However, there are many cases of severe injuries and even penile destructions caused by medical personnel in highly qualified centers.

According to the injured structure, penile injuries are classified into

- Penile skin loss
- Glans injury
- Meatal injury
- Urethral injuries
- Corporal injury
- Vascular injuries and ischaemia
- Penile amputation

EXCESSIVE PENILE SKIN LOSS

Wound dehiscence and degloving injuries of the shaft of the penis are possible following any of the techniques described before for neonatal circumcision, but it is generally more common with guillotine and free-handed methods and less common with the Gomco and Plastibell techniques. Degloving injuries usually result when an excess penile skin being drawn up into the clamp and then amputated or pulled distally the entire penile skin sheath and cutting it erroneously along the prepuce. Although, less likely, improper determination of the amount of skin to remove may occur during freehand circumcision.

From puberty on, penile bowing (curvature) and pain occur at the time of erection; skin loss is commonly seen at the ventral surface of the penis (Fig. 12.1); bizarre skin loss with disfigurement may result if a secondary infection supervenes, with resultant fibrosis and contracture that aggravate the situation (Fig. 12.2); and a circumferential skin loss is not rare, which complicates extensive preputial excision by unexperienced surgeon (Fig. 12.3).

Skin loss is also seen with other forms of penile injuries; as in the cases of ischaemic injuries and necrotizing fasciitis.

Excessive skin loss and degloving injuries may be diagnosed late secondary to extensive post-MC infection or after burn injury of the penile skin from thermal cautery (Fig. 12.4).

This complication is encountered mainly after circumcision of a congenitally abnormal penis as in the cases of webbed penis, microphallus, concealed penis and penis with a congenital chordee.

In webbed penis, if the surgeon tries to circumcise a baby by the classical method, like other normal babies, it will lead to extensive loss of the ventral skin (Fig. 12.1), so in such cases removal of the prepuce

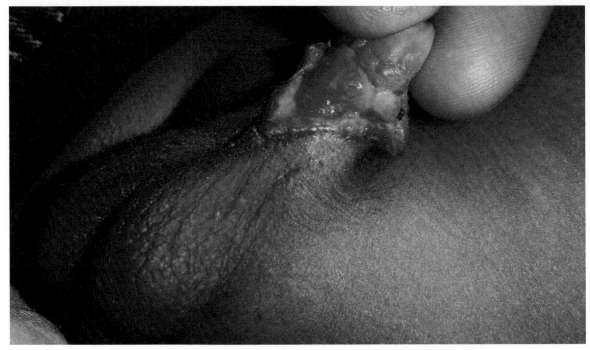

FIG. 12.1 Ventral skin loss after guillotine male circumcision of a webbed penis.

from the dorsum leaving only the ventral prepuce to cover the shaft with fine stitches may be enough, with an acceptable penile look. This simple method can be done by surgeons who had minimal experience with the different methods of flaps or V-Y plasty described in the literature for managing such cases. But sometimes, especially in severe cases, pedicled skin grafts or flaps are indicated.

Microphallus is another problem, as the circumciser may face some families that insist on doing circumcision early before the child can have an acceptable penile length, and in such cases, meticulous removal of a narrow strip of prepuce, making use of the rest of the prepuce to cover the shaft of the penis, may give acceptable results without skin loss.

Often these injuries are treated with an early local wound care and are allowed to heal by secondary intention, and later on, different local skin flaps can be utilized, such as lateral skin flaps (Fig. 12.5) or scrotal flaps, either in one or two stages (Fig. 12.6), but sometimes a free skin graft from the groin or other remote areas may be indicated.

GLANS INJURY

Glans injury may be seen as an isolated trauma, but it is commonly associated with meatal and urethral injuries. It is usually followed by attempts to stop bleeding of the glans wound by heavy haemostat or by using diathermy aggressively. Although many of such cases were detected immediately during the procedure, as it leads to extensive bleeding, but with prolonged tight compression dressing, glans injury may be discovered late (Fig. 12.7).

Necrosis of the glans can occur as a result of cautery injury during Gomco circumcision or from distal migration of an incorrectly sized Plastibell ring.[1]

Severe ischaemia or necrosis of the glans penis is rare, and it is commonly due to circumcision and trauma. Ischaemia of the glans penis following circumcision commonly results from dorsal penile nerve block with local anaesthetics and inadequate surgical technique or devices.[2]

Glans injury is not rare with the bone cutting guillotine method of MC. It is very rarely encountered with Gomco, Mogen and other clamps, which were designed entirely to protect the glans.

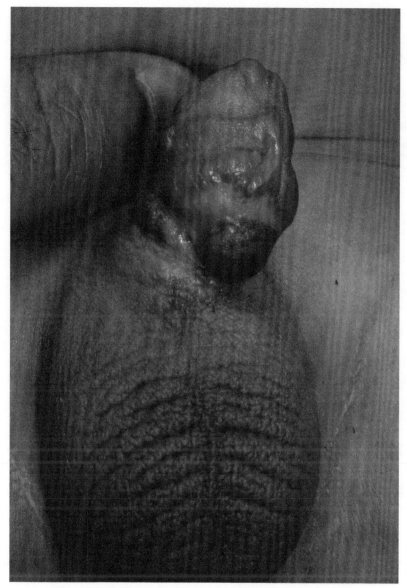

FIG. 12.2 Extensive fibrosis and contracture following skin loss.

Complete amputation of the glans occurs extremely rarely, but it is a devastating complication of Mogen clamp circumcision. This clamp seems uniquely susceptible to this particular injury given the surgeon's inability to directly visualize the glans before incising the foreskin.

Sequels of Glans Injury: Glans injury is commonly followed by:
- Meatal stenosis,
- Glandular fistula or glandular hypospadias (Fig. 12.8),
- Glans amputation and glandular disfigurement (Fig. 12.9).

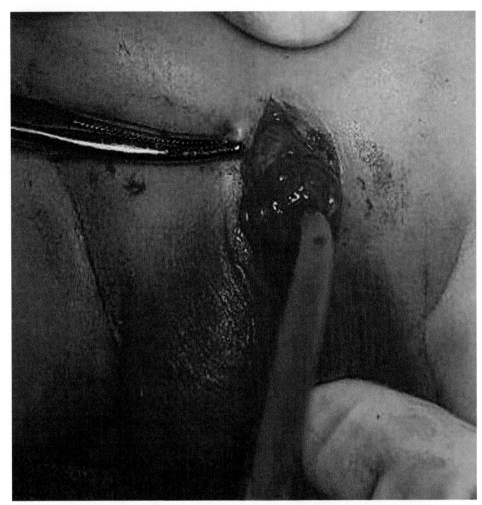

FIG. 12.3 Complete skin loss around the penis, extended to the suprapubic region.

MANAGEMENT OF GLANS INJURY

Prolonged compression immediately at the scene of circumcision may stop the bleeding. Bipolar diathermy could be utilized, but it should be used to stop the bleeding but it should be used at low current, and superficially, it is our policy to insert a fine catheter in all cases to avoid meatal stricture and urinary retention. Some authors reported management of severe cases with suprapubic urinary diversion and delayed urethroplasty, and a potent systemic antibiotic should be started to prevent any secondary infection.[2]

The main goal of treatment is to provide sufficient blood flow and deliver oxygen to the ischaemic penis. Pentoxifylline is a peripheral vasodilator and has been

shown to be beneficial in preventing ischaemic tissue damage accompanying various vascular diseases.

Late management should be tailored according to the residual defect, either repeated dilation for meatal stenosis or repair of the consequent hypospadias, but glans grafting usually provides unsatisfactory results (Fig. 12.10). Skeletonized, pedicled rectus abdominis muscle flap is an option for reconstruction of the amputated glans penis. Sherman et al. studied seven glandular reconstructions after traumatic amputations and reported that minimal debridement and recovery of the amputated tissue were critical to the repair. Simple primary reanastomosis of glandular tissue was possible in six of seven patients.[3] The patient's own tissue may

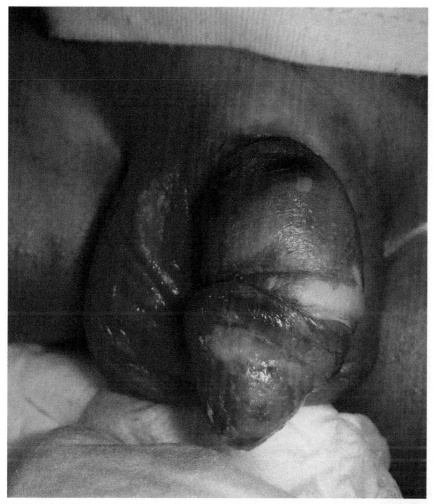

FIG. 12.4 Dorsal skin burning from the use thermal cauterization, sometimes healing may end with extensive fibrosis or skin loss.

remain viable up to 8 hours and can be used successfully for repair if adequately preserved by wrapping the tissue in moist saline gauze placed in a plastic bag and transported on ice.

MEATAL INJURY

Injury of the urinary meatus may be a direct traumatic mishap, or a secondary complication after balanitis or meatitis, with an incidence ranges between 10% and 20%.[2]

Direct meatal injury is not rarely seen after neonatal freehanded or nonmedical MC, either as an isolated minimal trauma or along glans injury. Many cases may not be recognized until late, when the mother notices a fine weak urinary stream or when the baby screams during micturition, such cases are difficult to differentiate from post-MC meatitis and stenosis, but a history of post-MC bleeding from the meatus, glans or frenulum and the use of diathermy to control it may refer to meatal injury (Fig. 12.11).

Repeated dilations may solve the problem in a majority of cases, but resistant or severe cases may need a meatoplasty.

POST-CIRCUMCISION URETHRAL INJURY
Urethrocutaneous Fistula (Iatrogenic Hypospadias)

Urethrocutaneous fistula is a rare complication, but nonetheless has been reported after all MC techniques.

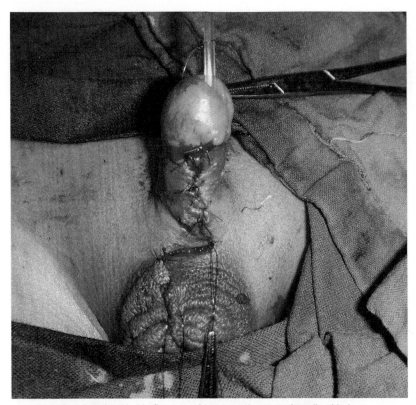

FIG. 12.5 Local skin flaps used to cover the ventral penile skin loss.

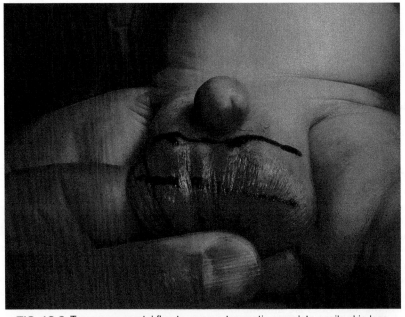

FIG. 12.6 Transverse scrotal flap to cover a traumatic complete penile skin loss.

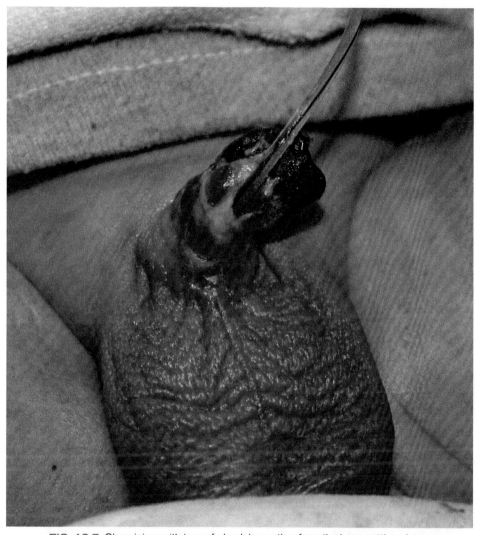

FIG. 12.7 Glans injury with loss of glandular urethra from the bone cutting clamp.

- Plastibell and Gomco circumcisions: Often this is a result of compression necrosis from a retained Plastibell ring or a direct injury from incorrect placement of the Gomco clamp. Isolated cases of fistula have been reported after the surgeon performed a ventral rather than a dorsal slit before initiation of circumcision.[4] It is important that the proper plane to be recognized for the initial lysis of adhesions so that the meatus is not inadvertently entered and then damaged (Fig. 12.12).

- Injury to the urethra during any ventral dissection can occur during a 'freehand' circumcision. Also urethral injury seems more likely to occur when there is bleeding from the frenulum and an attempt is made to control it with diathermy or a heavy suture. A suture placed too deeply that strangulates a part of the urethral wall or continuous application of high-current diathermy can lead to the formation of a fistula, which typically lies in the glans just proximal to the normal meatus at the site of the severed frenulum (Fig. 12.13).

- Extensive bacterial or mycotic urethritis after circumcision may also result in a proximal fistula, and extensive compression may contribute to tissue necrosis (Fig. 12.14). Our observation after collection of a considerable number of post-MC

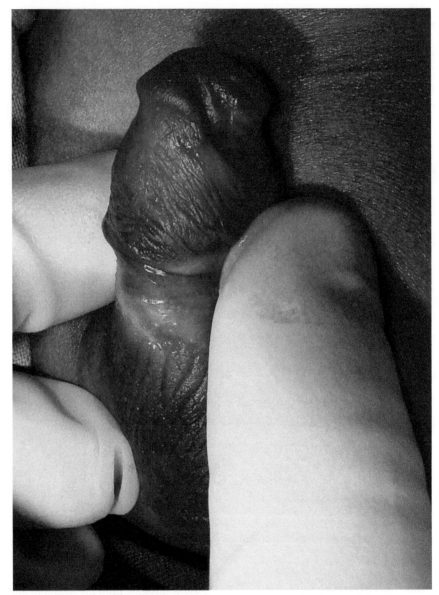

FIG. 12.8 Traumatic glandular hypospadias secondary to glans injury.

fistulae is that after infection and tissue necrosis, fistulae are usually detected away from the normal anatomic position of the urethra and even may be present at the root of the penis (Fig. 12.15), or dorsally, away from the urethral tract, (Fig. 12.16) with a relatively wide opening. Such fistulae develop weeks after a normal post-circumcision course, and to my knowledge, such varieties had not been reported before.

• Hair coil fistula: Bad hygiene, lack of follow-up and lack of supervision of the child after circumcision may lead to a disastrous fistula formation from a hair coil around the coronal sulcus. The hair coil fistula was reported in healthy babies without any relation to circumcision, but the healing circumcision wound is more liable to develop fistula after a hair coiling around or distal to the glans during the early post-circumcision period. This type of fistula is

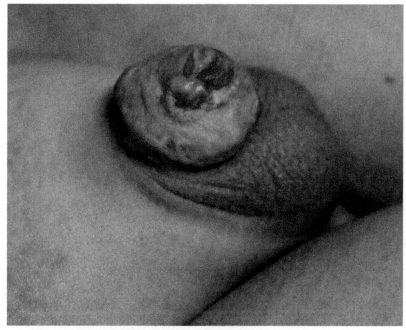

FIG. 12.9 Glandular disfigurement after glans injury.

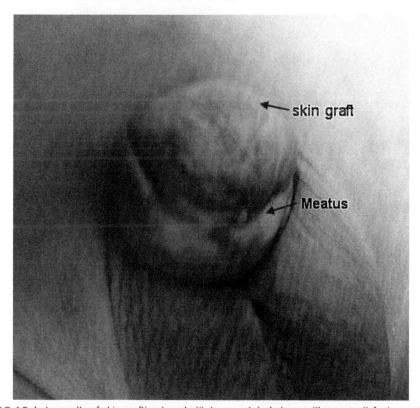

FIG. 12.10 Late results of skin grafting to substitute amputated glans, with an unsatisfactory outcome.

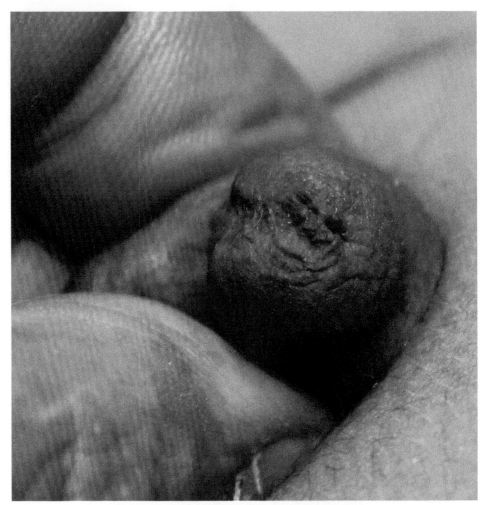

FIG. 12.11 Meatal stenosis secondary to meatal injury.

reported infrequently and is known as the penile tourniquet syndrome[5] (Fig. 12.17). Impaired blood supply to the area of coronal sulcus also leads to severe constriction of the sulcus, which may result in glandular atrophy or absorption (Fig. 12.18).

- While not technically a complication but a failure to recognize is the hypospadias or its variants [mainly megameatus intact prepuce (MIP)]. Those cases may be problematic both technically, as sometimes there is insufficient skin for the subsequent repair, and medicolegally, as the family may incriminate the circumciser as he is the one who induced this defect. Although most cases of hypospadias are associated with a dorsally hooded prepuce, the MIP variant will have a configuration to keep the penis looks normal

before preputial retraction. Thorough physical examination is imperative before attempting circumcision in order to detect any congenital anomalies, regardless of the method to be employed (Fig. 12.19). It is our trend to postpone any case of urethral or penile anomalies from the drift of cases coming for ritual MC. Median raphe anomalies may give the circumciser a clue about the presence of MIP anomaly before committing the circumcision.[6]

CLINICAL MANIFESTATIONS OF FISTULA COMPLICATIONS

Fistulae may present early after removal of the dressing or later on, after weeks, as an obvious fistulous tract or

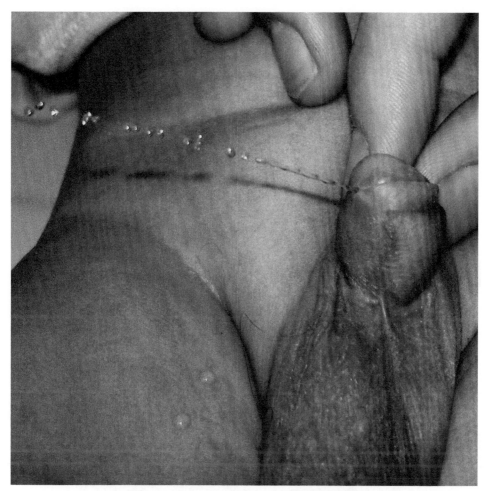

FIG. 12.12 A coronal fistula after Plastibell injury.

as a split urine stream (Fig. 12.20). Sometimes, especially in cases secondary to infection, a fistula may be presented firstly with a localized area of tissue necrosis or crusts and then becomes obvious as an abnormal opening. Most cases had combined injuries of the urethra and the glans or meatus.

MANAGEMENT

Fistula correction requires a second operation that is usually performed 6 months after the initial procedure. Repair of such cases is extremely difficult, with a high incidence of recurrence, so this fistula should be managed by an experienced hypospadiologist. At young age, a delayed flap repair can be done electively after the child's penis has grown enough for good tissue handling.

In attempting to repair such a fistula, it should be borne in mind that a circumcised penis has a little free skin available, particularly in the area of the frenum. The method chosen for repair should therefore be the safest. Urinary diversion and a repair without tension appear to be desirable.[7]

The prevention of fistula complications lies in the operators visualizing exactly what is being done in the course of a circumcision and includes family education and precise detection of any congenital anomalies before committing MC, with early referral of the patients who developed these complications to centres with paediatric urology experience.

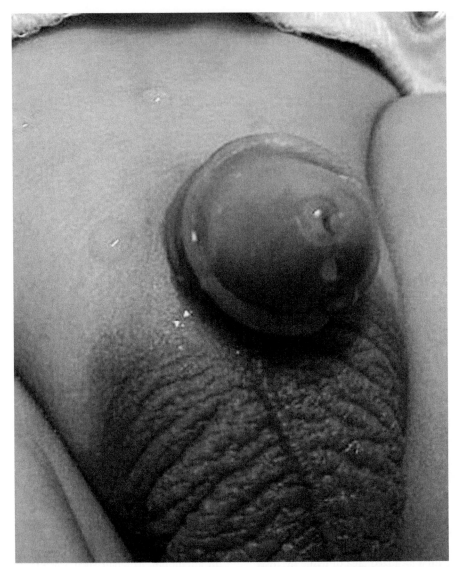

FIG. 12.13 A minute fistula proximal to the meatus secondary to the use of diathermy to control frenular bleeding.

CORPORAL INJURY

Corporal injury after MC is very rare, and it is manifested late as different grades of penile deviations. A few cases with corporal injuries had been reported, and it is difficult to presume this injury in as a complication after circumcision procedure, as it could be an undetected congenital anomaly that was just disclosed after MC.

Asymmetric congenital growth of the corpora, structural anomalies of dartos or a deficient tunica albuginea is responsible for the development of most cases of penile deviation.

Cases that may complicate MC may be secondary to a vascular insult compromising the corporal blood supply or tearing and rupturing of the tunica albuginea of the corpus cavernosum; these could be expected if there is a history of extensive dissection and if haematoma or oedema developed after circumcision (Fig. 12.21).

Penile rotation can cause psychosocial problems, painful intercourse and deviations in the urinary stream while standing (Fig. 12.22).

It is difficult to accurately estimate the incidence of such complications, as few cases are followed up strictly

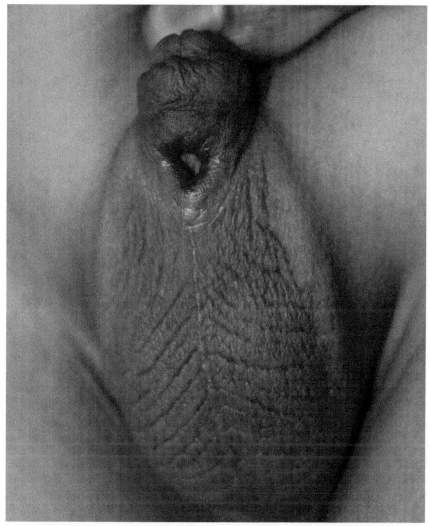

FIG. 12.14 A wide penoscrotal fistula developed 3 weeks after male circumcision in a normal 2-year-old boy.

after MC. In one retrospective study, penile rotation was diagnosed in 19 (3.2%) of 597 cases of neonatal circumcision.[8]

On the other hand, a chordee (a ventral curvature of the penis) may develop as a complication of circumcision. It is thought to be due to uneven amounts of foreskin removal from the ventral and dorsal surfaces, or due to different forms of adhesions and skin bridges. In this case, the corporal bodies are normally formed — unlike "true chordee" — but the healing of the asymmetric edge causes the glans to deviate.

Surgical correction may be necessary, with two major types of repair for congenital and acquired penile curvature: penile shortening and penile lengthening procedures. Penile shortening procedures include the Nesbit wedge resection and the plication techniques performed on the convex side of the penis. Penile lengthening procedures are performed on the concave side of the penis and require the use of a graft. Polat et al.[9] concluded that early surgical correction is possible, as tunica albuginea plication was also effective in prepubertal period.

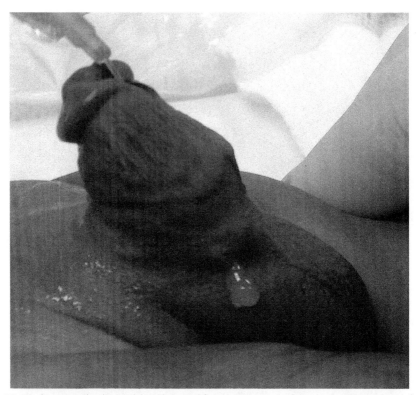

FIG. 12.15 A post-male circumcision abnormal fistula at the root of the penis with marked infection.

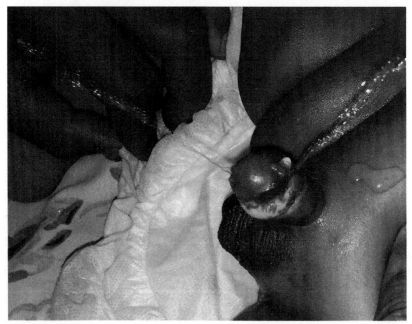

FIG. 12.16 Unreported case of a dorsal fistula in a neonate with a marked infection and necrosis seen well around the coronal sulcus after guillotine male circumcision.

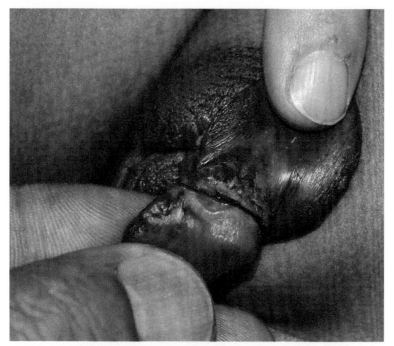

FIG. 12.17 A visible hair coil over the coronal sulcus in the early post-male circumcision period, resulting in a traumatic fistula.

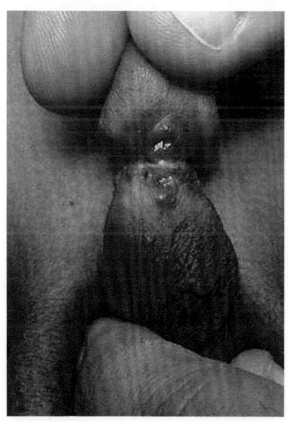

FIG. 12.18 Double fistulous openings with a degree of glandular atrophy after hair coil.

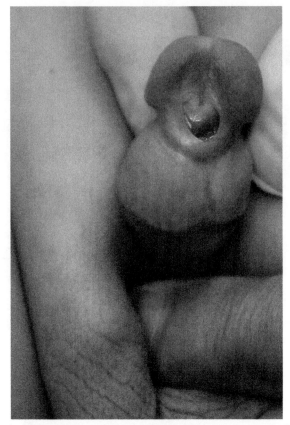

FIG. 12.19 A case of non recognized megameatus intact prepuce circumcised with a marked skin loss.

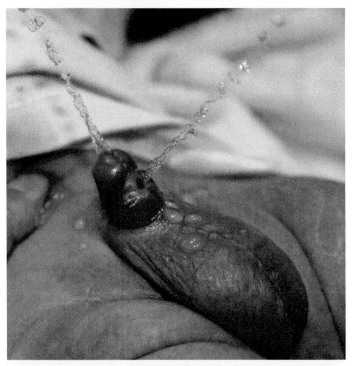

FIG. 12.20 An obvious fistula detected early after male circumcision.

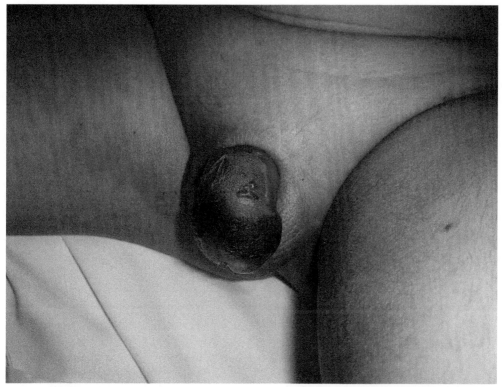

FIG. 12.21 Extensive penile haematoma after male circumcision, which may lead to corporal deficiency and rotation.

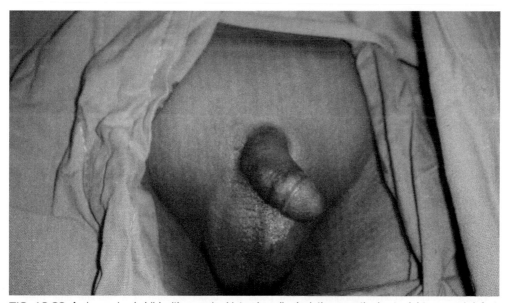

FIG. 12.22 A circumcised child with a marked lateral penile deviation, mostly due to right corporal defect.

VASCULAR INJURIES AND ISCHAEMIA

Necrosis and sloughing of the glans or even the entire penis has been reported after circumcision. Distal ischaemia with a subsequent tissue loss may result from infection, the use of anaesthetic solutions containing epinephrine, vigorous attempts at haemostasis with suture or cautery, prolonged use of a post-circumcision tourniquet or a tight bandage. Necrosis, in particular, is most likely to result if cautery is applied directly to a circumcision clamp (e.g. the Gomco clamp), with the use of unipolar or unearthed diathermy. When the entire penis is lost following such a mishap, a sequence of complications supervene the situation in the form of urethral stricture, retention of urine, proximal urinary tract obstruction and a horrific outcome.[10]

Fournier gangrene is a fulminant, spreading necrotizing infection of the skin and subcutaneous tissue of the scrotum, genitalia and/or perineum, which was first reported by Fournier in 1883.[11] Its cause may be identified in more than half of the cases. Incidence is around 1.6 cases per 100,000 men, with a mortality up to 20% −40% being reported in the past studies; however, recent reports show better outcome with mortality below 7.5%.[12]

Primary site affected is mostly the scrotum, due to minor abrasion or trauma, which then become progresses to the perineum, external genitalia and anterior abdominal wall. Primary isolated involvement of penis is very rare. It is rarely reported after circumcision, especially at older age, but this could also happen at a younger age, or even in a neonate, as we can see in Fig. 12.23, which shows a newborn with almost complete necrosis of the penis and upper part of scrotum after circumcision. Ischaemia and tissue necrosis may precede or predispose this severe infection.

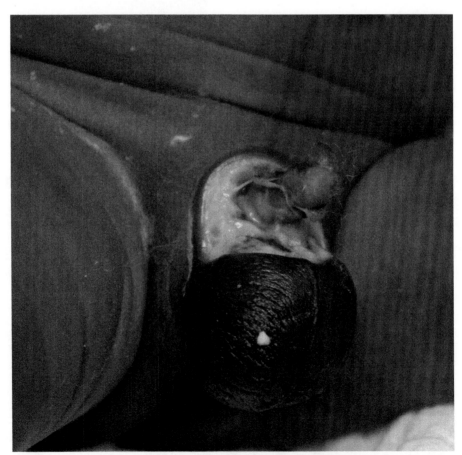

FIG. 12.23 Extensive Fournier gangrene of the penis and upper scrotum in a neonate after male circumcision.

The main pathologic in this condition is a polymicrobial infection with multiple aerobic and anaerobic bacteria. The primary pathophysiologic indication includes superficial necrosis due to arteriolar ischaemia, promoting further bacterial growth and rapid spread of infection. It remains a life-threatening disease that requires early recognition with aggressive surgical debridement, resuscitation and broad-spectrum antibiotics as the cornerstones of therapy.

In some situations, it may be extremely difficult to control penile ischaemia and to stop its proximal progression, with a subsequent sloughing of the glans or even the whole penis.

Treatment of Fournier gangrene of the penis is challenging. Urgent repeated debridement, with excision of all nonviable and necrotic tissues until well-perfused viable tissue is reached, and a proper antibiotic therapy is the key to successful management. Some authors reported a significant improvement after combining traditional surgical and antibiotic regimens with hyperbaric oxygen therapy (Chapter 13).[13]

Reconstruction, using scrotal flap or skin graft, gives excellent coverage, if the corpora and urethra remain intact, but cases of an ablatio penis will need phallic reconstruction.

PENILE ISCHAEMIA

Penis has a specially designed network of blood supply that protects this special organ from the usual causes of ischaemia, which affect the peripheral organs. Almost all cases of penile ischaemia are iatrogenic, with many factors that could contribute to compromising penile blood supply:

- Extensive combined infection, as in cases of Fournier gangrene,
- Extensive tissue destruction,
- Retained tight bandage after neonatal circumcision,
- Direct thermal injury of the penile blood vessels by monopolar diathermy or improper use of bipolar diathermy,
- Dorsal penile nerve block due to local anaesthesia infiltration with a vasoconstrictive agent.

Penile ischaemia may be manifested in a different spectrum:

- Ischaemia secondary to severing the frenular artery, either by different clamps or by heavy suturing; this usually a mild form of ischaemia, but may leads to meatal stenosis (Fig. 12.24).
- Ischaemia of the glans penis spreads down to the coronal sulcus with a normal penile shaft blood supply; this should be differentiated from glans

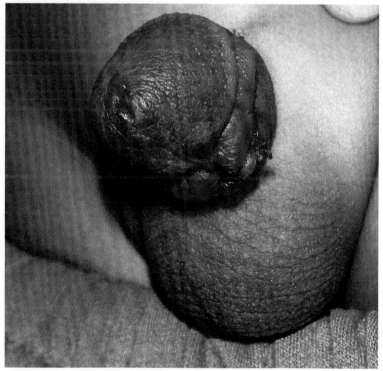

FIG. 12.24 Superficial ischaemia at the meatus secondary to heavy suturing of the frenular artery.

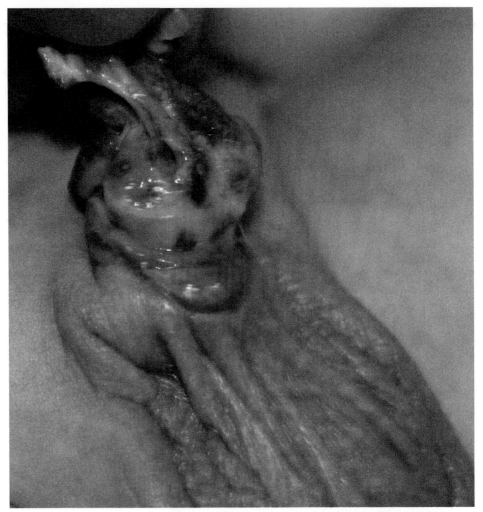

FIG. 12.25 Combined ischaemia and secondary penile infection, with glandular tissue loss.

injury (Fig. 12.7). In the former case, the glans contour is preserved with blackish discolouration. Glans ischaemia may affect the superficial layers only with a favourable outcome, or it may affect the deep tissues and result in glandular loss (Fig. 12.25).

- Whole penile shaft ischaemia and gangrene, which may lead to complete penile loss (aphallia) (Fig. 12.26).

MANAGEMENT

Cases with either glandular or penile ischaemia should be identified early and managed properly in a specialized centres, as an early combined use of intravenous pentoxifylline (which reduces blood viscosity, platelet aggregation and thrombus formation, and also acts as a powerful peripheral vasodilator) and hyperbaric oxygen was reported to improve some cases. The treatment will be less effective in cases detected late with an already detectable dry gangrene that has a line of demarcation[14] (Fig. 12.26).

Minimal or limited penile ischaemia, which does not affect all the blood supply of the penis, may respond well to pentoxifylline and hyperbaric oxygen therapy.[15] Figs. 12.27 and 12.28 show a case with distal ischaemia affecting only the glans penis that responded well to pentoxifylline injection and 16 daily sessions of hyperbaric oxygen with a favourable outcome.

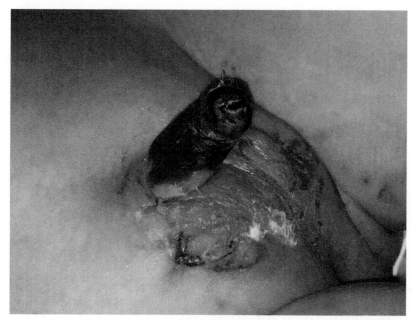

FIG. 12.26 Severe penile gangrene in a 4-year-old child after using monopolar diathermy for male circumcision, which was performed along another scrotal surgery.

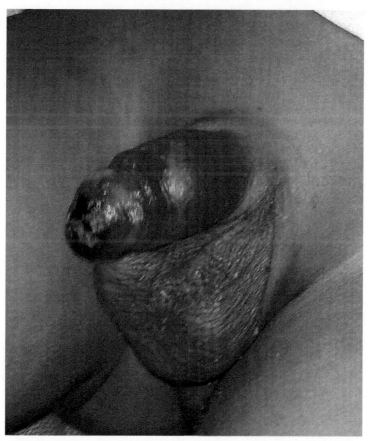

FIG. 12.27 A 2-year-old boy with glandular ischaemia 3 days after male circumcision.

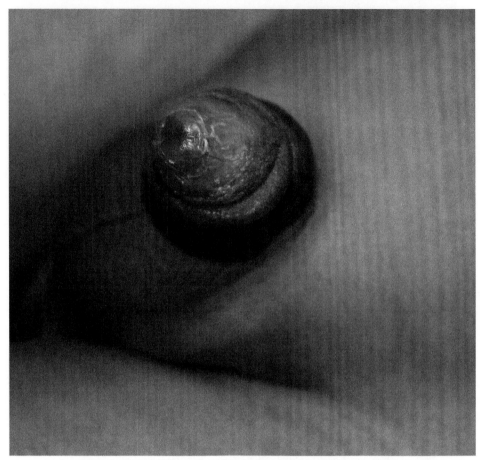

FIG. 12.28 Same child in Fig. 12.27 after 2 weeks of treatment with pentoxifylline and hyperbaric oxygen.

While phallic construction remains a challenging aspect of reconstructive surgery, penile transplantation has evolved tremendously during the past two decades, and a few cases had been attempted with some success in some centres.

In children with complete penile loss (ablatio penis), early management should be directed towards maintaining an adequate urine flow with an acceptable meatal calibre to avoid the need for urinary diversion, as well as to avoid urinary back pressure, stone formation and recurrent urinary tract infection (Fig. 12.29).

Children with complete penile loss face the option of either undergoing penile reconstruction with a forearm pedicle flap at adulthood or sex reassignment to female sex, which is another choice for neonates and young children.

PENILE AMPUTATION (GANGRENE AND PENILE LOSS)

The synonyms of penile amputation are penile denudation and ablation penis.

Penile amputation is fortunately rare after circumcision. The amputation may be partially glandular or partial to complete loss of the penis as a result of poor surgical technique, when the circumcision is performed by an unexperienced person in a traditional setting, or as a surgical mishap secondary to extensive penile ischaemia or Fournier gangrene (Fig. 12.23).

If not treated promptly, severe penile ischaemia may result in complete penile loss, with its sequels of urethral stenosis, stone formation and urinary back pressure with different grades of vesicoureteral reflux (Figs 12.29–12.31).

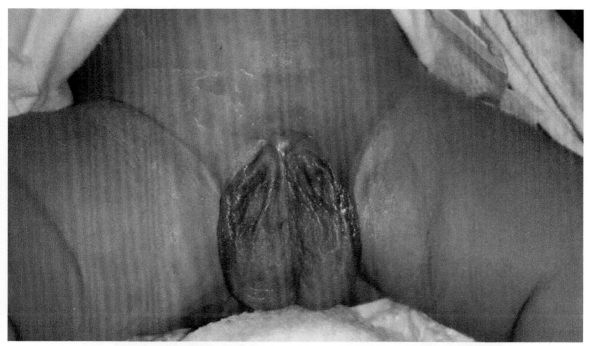

FIG. 12.29 Ablatio penis with a marked urethral stricture.

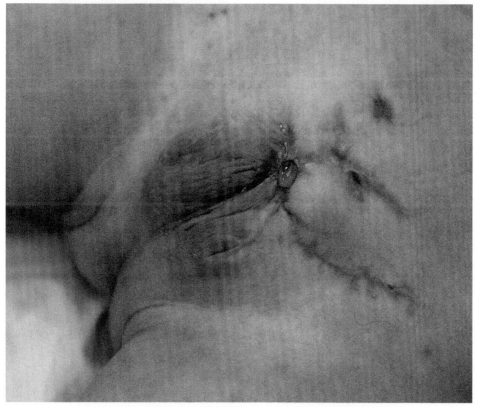

FIG. 12.30 Severe urethral stricture pursue complete penile loss.

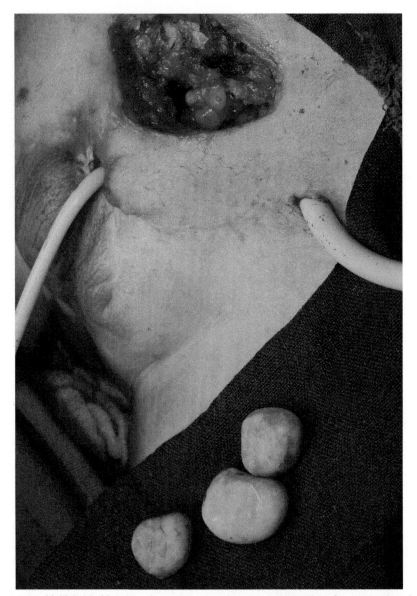

FIG. 12.31 Multiple bladder stone formation secondary to urine retention after traumatic aphallia.

Management

Glans and distal penile amputations may be treated as composite grafts by anastomosing the urethra and the corpora and then suturing the skin. These have been reported to be successful without microvascular anastomosis, with survival of the replanted penis depending upon the corporal sinusoidal blood flow; however, multiple complications are likely, including skin necrosis, venous congestion, urethral fistula or stricture, poor sensation and absent or incomplete erection. Ehrich[16]

reported successful replantation of an incompletely amputated penis by suturing the corpora and covering the denuded penis with scrotal skin, but the first microvascular replantation was reported by Cohen et al.[17] Microvascular replantation of the penis decreases the incidence of skin necrosis and other postoperative complications, but it is much more difficult in children because of the small size of the vessels.

Phalloplasty techniques are evolving to include a number of different flaps, and most techniques have high reported satisfaction rates. However, owing to the complexity of this procedure, it is not an ideal technique for every patient. Creation of a fully functional phallus remains elusive. Ideally, reconstruction of the penis should be completed in a single procedure and the reconstructed penis should be aesthetically acceptable, should retain erogenous and tactile sensation, should enable micturition while standing and should allow for penetrative sexual intercourse. Various operative techniques have been described, but given the lack of long-term efficacy and the potential morbidity of each technique, no ideal technique exists. Free radial forearm, abdominal, and anterolateral thigh flaps are the most studied and reported in the literature. In all techniques, complication rates are high, especially urethrocutaneous fistulae and stricture.

Penile replantation and transplantation are options for individuals with traumatic injuries, but only a few cases of penile transplants have been completed to date.[18]

REFERENCES

1. Gee WF, Ansell JS. Neonatal circumcision: a ten year overview: with comparison of the Gomco clamp and the Plastibell device. *Pediatrics*. 1976;58(6):824–827.
2. Sterenberg N, Golan J, Ben-Hur N. Necrosis of the glans penis following neonatal circumcision. *Plast Reconstr Surg*. 1981;68:237–239.
3. Sherman J, Borer JG, Horowitz M, Glassberg KI. Circumcision: successful glanular reconstruction and survival following traumatic amputation. *J Urol*. 1996;156(2): 842–844.
4. Bode CO, Ikhisemojie S, Ademuyiwa AO. Penile injuries from proximal migration of the Plastibell circumcision ring. *J Pediatr Urol*. 2010;6(1):23–27.
5. Badawy H1, Soliman A, Ouf A, Hammad A, Orabi S, Hanno A. Progressive hair coil penile tourniquet syndrome: multicenter experience with 25 cases. *J Pediatr Surg*. 2010;45(7):1514–1518. https://doi.org/10.1016/j.jpedsurg.2009.11.008.
6. Fahmy, et al. Penile median raphe anomalies as an indicator of megameatus intact prepuce anomaly in children undergoing routine circumcision. *Pediatric Urology*. 2018;121: 164–167. https://doi.org/10.1016/j.urology.2018.07.036. Available online 7 August 2018.
7. Niku D, Stock JA, Kaplan GW. Neonatal circumcision. *Urol Clin*. 1995;22(1):57–65.
8. Sakr A, et al. Complications of male circumcision over 10 years: single center experience. *Eur Urol Suppl*. 2017;16(3): e1061.
9. Polat EC, Erdem MR, Topaktas R, Ersoz C, Onol SY. Our experience in chordee without hypospadias: results of 102 cases. *Urol J*. 2014;11(4):1783–1787.
10. Pepe P1, Pietropaolo F, Candiano G, Pennisi M. Ischemia of the glans penis following circumcision: case report and revision of the literature. *Arch Ital Urol Androl*. 2015;87(1): 93–94. https://doi.org/10.4081/aiua.2015.1.93.
11. Woodside JR. Necrotizing fasciitis after neonatal circumcision. *Am J Dis Child*. 1980;134:301.
12. Chernyadyev, et al. Fournier's gangrene: literature review and clinical cases. *Urol Int*. 2018;101:91–97. https://doi.org/10.1159/000490108.
13. Gandhi J, et al. Clinical utility of hyperbaric oxygen therapy in genitourinary medicine. *Med Gas Res*. 2018;8(1): 29–33. https://doi.org/10.4103/2045-9912.229601.
14. Karaguzel E, Tok DS, Kazaz IO, et al. Postcircumcisional ischemia of the glans penis treated with Pentoxifylline. *Case Rep Urol*. 2013;2013:278523. https://doi.org/10.1155/2013/278523.
15. Migliorini F, Bianconi F, Bizzotto L, Porcaro AB, Artibani W. Acute ischemia of the glans penis after circumcision treated with hyperbaric therapy and Pentoxifylline: case report and revision of the literature. *Urol Int*. 2018; 100(3):361–363. https://doi.org/10.1159/000444399.
16. Ehrich WS. Two unusual penile injuries. *J Urol*. 1929;21: 239–241.
17. Cohen BE, May Jr JW, Daly JS, Young HH. Successful clinical replantation of an amputated penis by microneurovascular repair. Case report. *Plast Reconstr Surg*. 1977;59: 276–280.
18. Morrison SD, Shakir A, Vyas KS, Kirby J, Crane CN, Lee GK. Phalloplasty: a review of techniques and outcomes. *Plast Reconstr Surg*. 2016;138(3):594–615. https://doi.org/10.1097/PRS.0000000000002518.

CHAPTER 13

Role of Hyperbaric Oxygen Therapy in Male Circumcision Complications

AHMAD R. ABDEL-AAL, MS • MOHAMED A BAKY FAHMY, MD, FRCS

ABSTRACT

The field of hyperbaric oxygen therapy (HBOT) continues to develop and grow, and new indications are undergoing research and clinical trials. As this specialization evolves, more patients will benefit from improved techniques and protocols, broadening the scope with which HBOT is used. Research is ongoing around the world in areas that may benefit from HBOT, and it is our policy to use it for all cases of different grades of post-male circumcision penile ischaemia and in cases suspected or proved to have Fournier gangrene, as a supportive measure with other treatment modalities with satisfactory results. However, until now, our results and most of the other reports about the role of HBOT in penile injuries and deformities are observational.

KEYWORDS

Fournier gangrene; Hyperbaric oxygen; Penile ischaemia.

The innovation of hyperbaric therapy is one of the most interesting stories started about a century before the discovery of oxygen itself. Henshaw was the first to use alterations in atmospheric pressure for therapeutic purposes in 1662. He designed a chamber to treat chronic conditions with decreased pressure and acute diseases with increased pressure.[1] The discovery of oxygen is credited to Joseph Priestly in 1774, which he called it 'dephlogisticated air', and later named as 'oxygen' by Antoine Lavoisier. This led to advances not only in chemistry but also in the development of 'air baths' and oxygen chambers.[2]

In the early 1900s, Professor Cunningham noted that patients with heart disease did poorly at high altitudes and improved at sea level, which formed the basis for his use of hyperbaric air.[3] In 1918, he successfully treated patients of the Spanish influenza epidemic with hyperbaric air, and then he built the largest ever-constructed hyperbaric chamber (Fig. 13.1).

The field of hyperbaric oxygen treatment continues to develop and grow, and new indications are undergoing research and clinical trials. As this specialization evolves, more patients will benefit from improved techniques and protocols, broadening the scope with which hyperbaric oxygen therapy (HBOT) is used. Research is ongoing around the world in areas that may benefit from HBOT and controversies continue. Numerous diseases, conditions and syndromes have been treated with HBOT with varying levels of success; currently the Undersea and Hyperbaric Medical Society (UHMS) recognizes 14 major indications for the use of HBOT.[4]

One of the dangers unique to HBOT was the potential for decompression sickness, but barotrauma and arterial gas embolism in hyperbaric rooms are the most serious complications. The main predisposing factors for complications after HBOT, which should be avoided, are dehydration, obstructed middle ear, otitis media, flying after a hyperbaric dive and heavy exercise; many safety measures were proposed to reduce these risks.

For patients with an underlying ischaemic process, HBOT is considered as a supplemental treatment, in addition to the conventional surgical and medical approaches in different pathologic conditions, generally for facilitating acute wound healing. Its role is mainly reported in penile diseases as a treatment of perineal necrotizing fasciitis (Fournier gangrene) and for post-traumatic penile ischaemic injuries following circumcision at different age groups.

At sea level, most oxygen in the blood is inside the red blood cells (RBCs) and little oxygen dissolves in plasma (<3 mL). Oxygen levels in plasma (liquid portion) can be increased with pressure according to Henry's law, which will result in increased tissue oxygenation.

Complications in Male Circumcision. https://doi.org/10.1016/B978-0-323-68127-8.00013-2

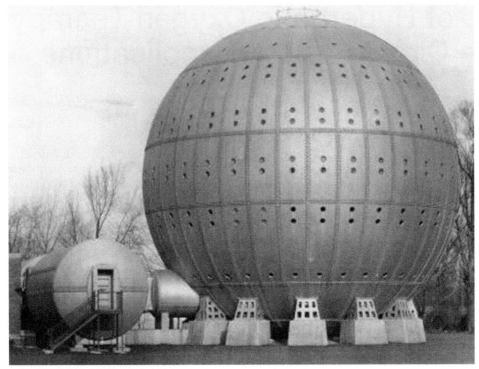

FIG. 13.1 The largest hyperbaric chamber in the world that was constructed a few years after the end of the First World War in Cleveland, Ohio, USA.

At normal atmospheric pressure, the arterial oxygen tension is about 100 mmHg and tissue oxygen tension is about 55 mmHg. But when pressure is increased threefold as in HBOT, 100% oxygen can increase the arterial oxygen tension to 2000 mmHg and tissue oxygen tension to around 500 mmHg. This leads to a rise in dissolved oxygen concentration from 3 mL/L to 60 mL/L, which is the concentration a normally perfused tissue requires. The delivery of 60 mL oxygen per litre of blood is enough for the plasma oxygen to reach the obstructed areas of resting tissues, where RBCs cannot reach and without the need for oxygen carried by their haemoglobin.[5]

HBOT improves wound healing by amplifying oxygen gradients along the periphery of ischaemic wounds; it also promotes oxygen-dependent collagen matrix formation needed for angiogenesis.[6]

HBOT also enhances the production of oxygen free radicals, which oxidize proteins and membrane lipids, destruct DNA and decrease bacterial metabolism. It also facilitates the oxygen-dependent peroxidase system by which leucocytes kill bacteria. Also the mode of action of hyperbaric oxygen (HBO) may be through optimal tissue oxygenation, which potentiates or restores the host's bactericidal mechanisms and wound healing activity in patients who suffered from serious synergetic aerobic and anaerobic infections of the cutaneous and subcutaneous tissues; it is proved that HBOT has a direct toxic effect on anaerobic bacteria.[7]

Moreover, HBOT improves the oxygen-dependent transport of certain antibiotics across bacterial cell walls.[8]

Zhong et al.[9] reported a case with successful engraftment and function by combining a microsurgical procedure and postoperative supplemental care with HBOT, which was used to accelerate the healing process. Similar success was reported by Faydaci et al.[10] for a case of glans penis amputation as a rare circumcision complication.

It is our policy to use HBO in all cases of different grades of post-male circumcision (MC) penile ischaemia and in cases suspected or proved to have Fournier gangrene as a supportive measure with other treatment modalities (Fig. 13.2). Cases diagnosed with different grades of only penile ischaemia, with or without thermal injuries after MC, are managed with pentoxifylline infusion and sequential daily HBOT till appreciation

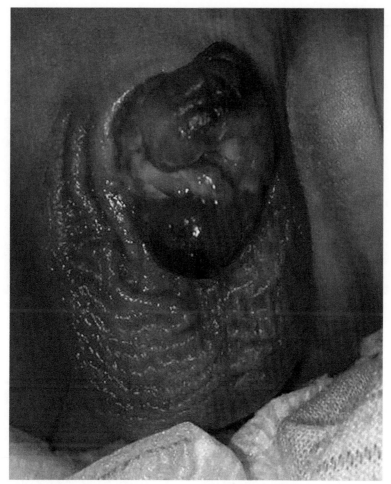

FIG. 13.2 Infant with post-male circumcision ischaemia associated with microbial infection and tissue necrosis.

of improvement and good tissue perfusion (usually after 3−4 weeks), with excellent results in all cases (Fig. 13.3).

We have a specially designed HBO cabinet designed for neonates and infants, with gradual pressure increment till reaching 1.4 barometric pressure (760 mmHg) for 20 min, and after that oxygen is given for 1 hour daily for 5 days per week. Older children are managed in the conventional HBO chamber with the same regimen (Fig. 13.4).

A few cases with post-MC corporal injury and cases with different grades of urethral fistula are managed with HBO for 2−3 weeks before commencing surgical correction with satisfactory results, but till now, our results and most of the other reports about the role of HBO in penile injuries and deformities are observational. Müller et al.[11] conducted a study to define the effects of HBOT on erectile function (EF) and cavernosal tissue in the rat cavernous nerve (CN) injury model, and they concluded that HBOT following a CN injury, improving EF preservation in this model and supporting the cavernosal oxygenation concept as a protective mechanism for EF. The effects appear to be mediated via preservation of neurotrophic and endothelial factor expression.

A controlled randomized study is required to prove the role of HBO in the management of ischaemic injury of the genitalia and to compare its effect with other treatment modalities, but this is not an easy task. Also, research and randomized clinical trials continue in several areas of medicine, which are not yet recognized as indications for HBOT.

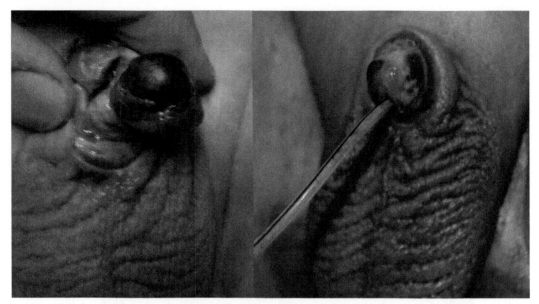

FIG. 13.3 A case of post-male circumcision ischaemic injury before and after giving hyperbaric oxygen therapy for 3 weeks.

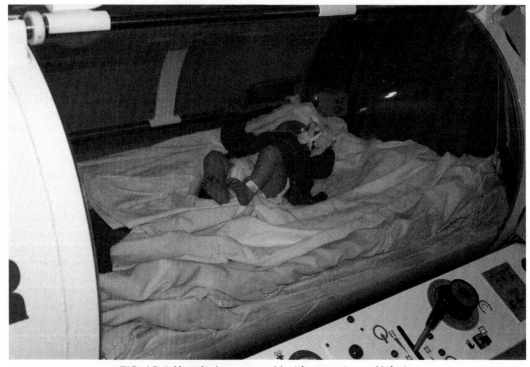

FIG. 13.4 Hyperbaric oxygen cabinet for neonates and infants.

REFERENCES

1. Simpson A. *Compressed Air, as a Therapeutic Agent in the Treatment of Consumption, Asthma, Chronic Bronchitis, and Other Diseases*. Edinburgh, Scotland: Sutherland and Knox; 1857.

2. Williams KR. The discovery of oxygen and other Priestley matters. *J Chem Educ*. 2003;80(10):2003.

3. Cunningham OJ. Oxygen therapy by means of compressed air. *Anesth Analg*. 1927;6:64.

4. Carney AY. Hyperbaric oxygen therapy an introduction. *Crit Care Nurs Q*. 2013;36(No. 3):274−279. https://doi.org/10.1097/CNQ.0b013e318294e936.

5. Leach RM, Rees PJ, Wilmshurst P. Hyperbaric oxygen therapy. *Br Med J*. 1998;317:1140−1143.

6. Hunt TK. The physiology of wound healing. *Ann Emerg Med*. 1988;17:1265−1273.

7. Xie, et al. The role of hyperbaric oxygen therapy in andrology. *Int Arch Urol Complic*. 2017;3:022. https://doi.org/10.23937/2469-5742/1510022.

8. Knighton DR, Halliday B, Hunt TK. Oxygen as an antibiotic: the effect of inspired oxygen on infection. *Arch Surg*. 1984;119:199−204.

9. Zhong Z, Dong Z, Lu Q, Li Y, Lv C, et al. Successful penile replantation with adjuvant hyperbaric oxygen treatment. *Urology*. 2007;69:983.

10. Faydaci G, Ugur K, Osman C, Sermin S, Bilal E. Amputation of glans penis: a rare circumcision complication and successful management with primary anastomosis and hyperbaric oxygen therapy. *Korean J Urol*. 2011;52:147−149.

11. Müller A, Tal R, Donohue JF, Akin-Olugbade Y, Kobylarz K, et al. The effect of hyperbaric oxygen therapy on erectile function recovery in a rat cavernous nerve injury model. *J Sex Med*. 2008;5:562−570.

CHAPTER 14

Prevention of Male Circumcision Complications

MOHAMED A BAKY FAHMY, MD, FRCS

ABSTRACT

Away from the debate between scholars who recommend or fight against male circumcision, the magnitude of complications following this very common procedure is alarming, and the procedure requires a workup to prevent and to manage properly and timely any detectable complication. The most important points — in my opinion — are the guidelines for safe procedure and a scheduled long-term follow-up. Links between the formal and informal health sectors should be explored elsewhere to institute quality standard practices for both traditional and medical circumcisers, for example, wearing sterile gloves, using sterile instruments and appropriate after-care, and for creating a formal structure to monitor and regulate the conduct of circumcision.

KEYWORDS

Guidelines; Prevention.

Away from the debate between scholars who recommend or fight against male circumcision, the magnitude of complications following this very common procedure is alarming, and the procedure requires a workup to prevent and to manage properly and timely any detectable complication. The most important points — in my opinion — are the guidelines for safe procedure and a scheduled long-term follow-up.

Links between the formal and informal health sectors should be explored elsewhere to institute quality standard practices for both traditional and medical circumcisers, for example, wearing sterile gloves, using sterile instruments and appropriate after-care, and for creating a formal structure to monitor and regulate the conduct of circumcision. Through these steps, it is likely that the safety of this common procedure can be substantially improved.

There is a lack of a standardized operating practice for circumcision, including the management and reporting of adverse events. Further prospective studies of circumcision risks are needed, with rigorous documentation using standardized definitions, to compare the relative risks of different methods, to identify the optimal age for circumcision and to study the impact of specific and ongoing training of providers.

Unacceptable levels of risk have been recorded in some prospective studies of child circumcision by medical providers, and there is an urgent need to improve the safety of the procedure through renewed training where necessary. Setting-specific strategies for such training are needed, including guidelines for safe neonatal and child circumcision, both in settings where it is conducted already and in those where it may be introduced for HIV prevention.

The risks following the traditional circumcision of older boys tend to be even higher and are a cause of unnecessary morbidity. Methods to improve training and practices are urgently needed in order to avoid unnecessary morbidity and could follow the examples of the good links between the formal and informal healthcare services for the provision of traditional neonatal circumcision in developing countries.

The use of anaesthesia for circumcision varies widely, with general anaesthesia common in infant circumcision in the United States, local anaesthesia used in other settings and no anaesthesia used in most other places, especially for traditional circumcision. Local anaesthesia for neonatal and infant circumcision is recommended by the WHO, and there is a need to improve the training of circumcision providers in order to educate them on the appropriate methods of anaesthesia and hygiene practices.

A number of new devices are now available that are suitable for the circumcision of men of all ages, from infancy to adulthood. To date, there is little published data on the performance of these devices, and detailed

Complications in Male Circumcision. https://doi.org/10.1016/B978-0-323-68127-8.00014-4

reviews and comparisons of safety, cost and client satisfaction are needed.

Neonatal and child circumcision is routinely practised in many countries for religious, cultural or medical reasons. The procedure is undertaken by a range of providers, with the choice of provider depending on family or religious tradition, cost, availability and perception of service quality. As a traditional religious and cultural practice, circumcision is likely to continue to be highly prevalent around the world and, in addition, is now being considered for HIV prevention. Every effort must be made to ensure that the procedure is undertaken as safely as possible by trained and experienced providers with adequate supplies and in hygienic conditions.

A set of guidelines on the expansion of circumcision services produced by the WHO and UNAIDS (Joint United Nations Programme on HIV/AIDS) includes operational guidance for scaling up circumcision for HIV prevention, a surgical manual for circumcision under local anaesthesia, guidance for decision makers on human rights and ethical as well as legal considerations for protocols for monitoring and evaluation.

There is a clear need to improve the safety of circumcision in all ages through improved training or retraining for both traditional and medically trained providers and to ensure that providers have adequate supplies of the necessary equipment and instruments for safe circumcision. Strategies for training and quality assurance are needed and will be context specific. In Swaziland, Operation AB demonstrated a comprehensive model of training teams of medical providers in safe and swift adolescent and adult circumcisions, with improved sterilization equipment and client education, at community-level clinics.[1]

In Ghana, where neonatal circumcision is almost universal, the formal health service provides training to traditional providers in Accra, with training on basic hygiene and the provision of necessary equipment, such as sterile gloves and dressings.

In South Africa, it has been suggested that community health nurses create opportunities to educate traditional circumcisers of adolescents and adults on the basic hygiene requirements to be met before, during and after circumcision.[2]

The British Association of Paediatric Surgeons suggests that circumcision be performed only by those who can perform the procedure, recognize any comorbidity and complications and have access to medical care should complications arise.[3]

REFERENCES

1. *Operation Abraham*; 2008. http://www.operation-ab.org/.
2. Mayatula V, Mavundla TR. A review on male circumcision procedures among South African blacks. *Curationis*. 1997; 20(3):16–20.
3. *British Association of Paediatric Surgeons Guidelines*. http://www.baps.org.uk/documents/RELCIRC.html.

CHAPTER 15

Reconstructive Surgery for Circumcision Complications

MOHAMED A BAKY FAHMY, MD, FRCS

ABSTRACT

Reconstructive remedy of the consequent complications after male circumcision, especially during childhood, is well described in the late 1980s by illustrious predecessors; however, during the past 10 years, both medical and surgical treatment strategies had advanced enough to raise patient expectations for better long-term outcomes. As a child with complications of circumcision grew into adulthood, it became apparent that the results of many early interventions by pediatric urologists were not as good as originally hoped for, especially when the patient is exposed to scrutiny by his partner or when the patients compare themselves to normalcy.

Challenge is clear in cases of multiple complications, and failure is usually clear when the reconstructive surgeons failed to recognize the normally anthropometric appearance of the aesthetic penis and to achieve normalization of function. Circumcision complications are commonly seen in men who had formerly minor or nondetectable penile congenital anomalies such as webbed penis, microphallus, microposthia, penile chordee and rotational anomalies. Such complications had a wide range of diversity and severity and there is no unified surgical procedure described specifically for such cases; each complication deserves a technique tailored for every patient, but general reconstructive principles are applicable for dealing with circumcision sequels.

Phalloplasty techniques, for cases of post-circumcision penile loss, are evolving to include a number of different flaps, and most techniques have high reported satisfaction rates. Penile replantation and transplantation are also options for amputation or loss of phallus. Further studies are required to better compare different techniques to more robustly establish best practices.

KEYWORDS

Foreskin regeneration; Foreskin restoration; Penile visibility index; Phalloplasty; Posthioplastice; Preputioplasty.

GENERAL PRINCIPLES OF RECONSTRUCTION OF COMPLICATIONS AFTER MALE CIRCUMCISION

- Children or adults who were subjected to circumcision, whatever its indication, should not carry any consequence throughout their life, even if only a surgical scar.
- Penile injuries are best treated by experienced surgeons on a case-by-case basis, with care taken to identify the most appropriate treatment.
- Every circumciser should be trained to have a setting of expectations and eventual aesthetic satisfactory outcomes for their patients.
- Excessive inner or outer prepuce is not an indication for redoing circumcision, and if the family or the patient himself insisted on refashioning, it is not considered a reconstructive surgery.
- Early intervention is not advisable, except in cases that need life or organ saving. The only advantage of neonatal and infancy intervention is prevention of subsequent psychic trauma; otherwise, late intervention is recommended for proper planning of the reconstruction and appropriate tissue handling.
- Skin grafting of the penis can be challenging because of the ability of the penis to change in size.
- Local penile tissue is the best material for reconstruction as a flap, followed by scrotal skin, but if the skin in these areas is deficient, then a groin or upper thigh free graft is the second choice.[1]
- Owing to the dramatic change in the size of the penis during erection and the need for durability because of the tissue demands of sexual activity, full-thickness skin grafts seem to be the preferred choice for the replacement of penile skin. However, in most cases, penile skin is best replaced by a split-thickness skin graft. A thick split-thickness skin graft offers the best combination of graft take and durability.[2]

Complications in Male Circumcision. https://doi.org/10.1016/B978-0-323-68127-8.00015-6

- In some cases, a full-thickness skin graft may be appropriate in penile reconstruction. The most common example is in urethral reconstruction. Although a detailed discussion of graft urethroplasty is outside the scope of this chapter, understanding the principles behind graft selection and the factors that determine success is essential. Urethral reconstruction requires tissue that resists the stress of urine passage. At present, a full-thickness oral mucosal graft is the closest replacement tissue for the urethra. It is used extensively in staged reconstruction of urethral repairs and complex hypospadias.[3]

PREPUTIAL RECONSTRUCTION

Synonyms: Foreskin restoration, posthioplastice, uncircumcision, decircumcision or posthioplasty.

Definition: Foreskin restoration involves covering the glans penis to some extent with a double sheath of retractable tissue.

The demand for surgical or nonsurgical restoration of the prepuce after circumcision was so old that even the first evidence for such a procedure is mentioned in the Bible. Celsus (25 BCE to CE 50) and Galen (CE 131—200) have given a detailed description on how to restore the foreskin in circumcised persons. The first detailed description of an operative procedure for decircumcision was given by Celsus, as seen in Fig. 15.1.

Nowadays, reports on surgical foreskin restoration are still rare and alternative methods of nonsurgical skin expansion have become more common. With progressive decline in the rate of ritual circumcision in many countries, several organizations were founded to give advice on and support to foreskin restoration, such as the National Organization of Restoring Men (NORM). http://www.norm.org/.

Different methods and techniques are available to restore the foreskin in adults who regret after male circumcision and look for restoration of the removed prepuce, with all the procedures aiming to provide an extra single layer of skin to cover the glans. However, the only hope to regain a structure similar to the unique prepuce with its complicated components is through tissue engineering to reconstruct a new prepuce (preputial cloning), with promising results, but it is still an expensive procedure.

Preputial restoration could be achieved via nonsurgical and surgical procedures.

Nonsurgical Restoration
Skin expansion
Modern techniques of stretching penile skin have become famous only as lately as in the 1980s. Today, foreskin stretching is widely performed in the United States, and all methods depend on some kind of tape that is attached to the skin. The easiest way to start with is to pull the residual foreskin or the skin of the penile shaft over the glans as far as possible. The skin is fixed in this position by one or two tape straps that run from one side of the stretched penile skin over the tip of the glans to the other side of the shaft. If there is enough foreskin to cover the whole glans, it is also possible to apply a tape ring around the distal skin of the new prepuce that makes it impossible to retract. The tape is either changed daily or, in most cases, left until it gets off the skin. In these simple methods, simple pressure from the glans will start stretching the skin.[4]

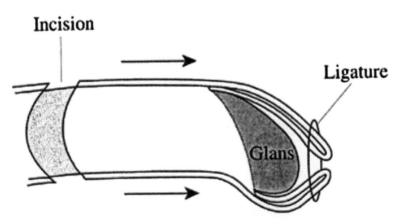

FIG. 15.1 Celsus' first method of "decircumcision," with distal circumferential cutting of the penile skin and proximal pulling of the skin to cover the glans. (After Rubin JP. Celsus' decircumcision operation. Urology. 1980;16:121.)

Unlike conventional skin expansion techniques, the process of nonsurgical foreskin restoration may take several years to complete. The time required depends on the amount of skin available to expand, the amount of skin desired in the end and the regimen of stretching methods used. Patience and dedication are needed and there are support groups to help with these; the act of stretching the skin is often described informally as "tugging" by the support groups, especially those on the Internet.[5]

Several commercial retaining devices are available to hold the remaining skin. Tissue expansion cannot restore the specialized structures, and it is unclear whether the process promotes any nerve regeneration. Nonsurgical tissue expansion methods are state of the art, as they produce a pseudo-foreskin with much higher cosmetic appearance and functionality than that produced by surgical methods; also they are far less expensive; and do not have an associated risks as surgical methods.

Older methods have been partially replaced by the use of various plastic or silicone components. The entire design and function of the 'modern' devices were first described in 2003 (Fig. 15.2).

Many new devices grip the skin, usually without the use of a tape. Some devices are homemade, often designed by men whose skin is easily irritated by adhesive tapes, also there are several different varieties of tapeless restoration devices commercially available.

In some cases where there is too little skin to pull onto the gripping surface, pressure must be applied to the glans when applying the device. Most devices and weights are easily washed and can be reused each day.

Excessive tension may cause scar tissue to form, which takes longer to 'heal' and hinders flexibility of the newly acquired skin. It is important to perform pressure tests to check the blood flow. Furthermore, as part of the restoration regimen, no matter what device is being used, there must be frequent release of the tension against the sheath tissue and/or pressure against the glans so as to allow for free blood circulation.

Surgical Restoration

Surgical reconstruction methods include the following:

1. Skin graft from the thigh or buttocks: A free skin graft is sutured into a circumferential cut made around the penile shaft at the circumcision scar. The transplanted tissue usually has a very different condition and texture and is quite inflexible and smooth.
2. Scrotal implant flap: A scrotal implant graft is a multiple-stage reconstruction, involving circumferentially cutting the shaft tissue at the circumcision scar. A tunnel is created in the front side of the scrotum between two incisions and then the penile shaft is threaded through the tunnel and stitched at both ends. After about 3−6 months, when healed, the penis is surgically removed with the new scrotal tissue cut on either side and wrapped around the shaft and sewn on the ventral side. There is then another healing period. At that point, it is typically necessary to reduce the 'overhang' and to enlarge the orifice of the new foreskin.
3. Z-plasty or Y-V plasty: It is used to lengthen the distal penile skin to cover the glans partially.

Foreskin regeneration

There has been remarkable success in the field of regenerative medicine in the past two decades. There has been growing interest to regenerate the human male foreskin, and many clinical trials registered for regeneration of the human prepuce.

The proposed method would involve placing the patient under general anaesthesia. The penile skin would be opened at the circumcision scar, which is surgically derided. A biomedical solution would then be applied to both ends of the wound, causing the foreskin to regenerate with the DNA in the patient's cells. A biodegradable scaffold (i.e., the decellularized foreskin of a cadaver) would be used to offer support for the regenerating foreskin. In the United States, Purpura et al.[6] developed an innovative, regenerative therapy to repair the lost foreskin through the development of biological, acellular scaffolds by using decellularized foreskin dermal matrices, which prove to be able to maintain a balance between cellular removal and the maintenance of structural, mechanical and biological properties of the foreskin tissue.

Preputioplasty

The term preputioplasty is a misleading one because it is used only to describe the limited dorsal slit with transverse closure, which is used for surgical management of phimosis as a substitution for circumcision. Preputioplasty is used to widen a narrow nonretractile foreskin that cannot be comfortably drawn back off the head of the penis during erection because of a constriction (stenosis) that has not expanded after adolescence, so it is not related to preputial reconstruction (PR).

The dorsal slit, as traditionally and still occasionally performed, is rarely to be recommended because the cosmetic result is unsatisfactory, longitudinal incision of the constricting ring proximal to the preputial

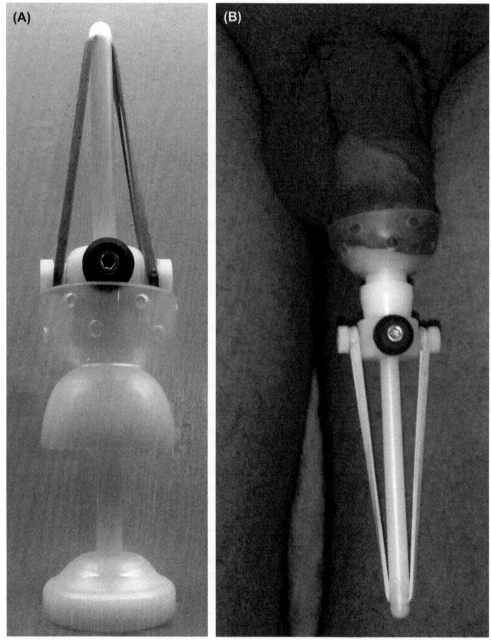

FIG. 15.2 **(A)** Dual tension restorer (DTR, tapeless device) **(B)** applied to a circumcised penis for foreskin restoration.

meatus, again with transverse suture as another alternative. Dean et al.[7] developed a geometric variant of the dorsal slit procedure by adding a ventral slit to achieve the natural appearance of an intact foreskin and to be easily fully retractable (Fig. 15.3).

Lane and South[8] described lateral preputioplasty as a variant of the dorsal slit. In this procedure, two laterally placed longitudinal incisions were made and the defects were sutured transversely. The authors advocated that the lateral placement of the incisions provides cosmetic

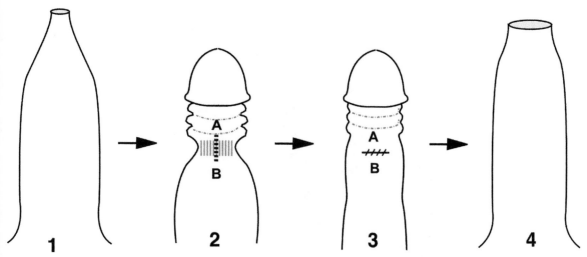

FIG. 15.3 (1) Penis with a tight phimotic ring making it difficult to retract the foreskin. (2) Foreskin retracted under anaesthesia, with the phimotic ring or stenosis constricting the shaft of the penis and creating a 'waist'. (3) Incision closed laterally. (4) Penis with the loosened foreskin replaced over the glans.

improvement over the dorsal approach and avoids the impairment of frenular area over circumcision or other procedures, including ventral slits.

A triple-incision preputioplasty was described by Welsh in 1936. The technique consisted of three longitudinal, full-thickness skin incisions across the stenotic ring down to the inner preputial layer and transversal suturing of the three defects to enlarge a phimotic ring (Fig. 15.4). Wåhlin[9] modified the procedure and three rhomboid defects made by the longitudinal incisions were closed with interrupted sutures placed obliquely in the middle of each incision.

Nonsurgical technique is now available to manage phimosis by widening the tight prepuce without surgery; a speculum can be inserted into the phimotic foreskin and it puts tension in a lateral direction to gently open the foreskin so that it will allow retraction over the glans, with time, new cells are formed and the opening widens.[10]

Preputial reconstruction in hypospadias surgery

In hypospadias surgery the prepuce can be reconstructed, but the procedure has not gained wide acceptance in all centers, and PR is surrounded by several controversies.

PR can be important for some patients or their parents, and it can be performed in almost all patients with distal hypospadias, except perhaps in those with the most asymmetric prepuces or severe ventral skin

deficiency. PR does not seem to increase urethroplasty complications, but combination of PR with tubularization of the urethral plate urethroplasty seems to offer the best chance of success. Specific complications occur in around 8% of patients and include partial or complete dehiscence of the prepuce and secondary phimosis. To prevent the latter, the reconstructed prepuce should be easily retractile at the end of surgery. Technical modifications can help achieve this goal. Cosmetically, reconstructed prepuces are not fully normal, but the abnormality could be less important for a patient and his parents than the complete absence of the prepuce.[11]

Preputial oedema and lymphoedema is common in PR after hypospadias surgery, but most cases are self-limited and respond to conservative measures (Fig. 15.5).

PENILE ROTATION

The pathogenesis of penile torsion lies in the eccentric fusion of the endodermal and/or ectodermal folds. This leads to misdirected mesodermal proliferation during formation of the corpora and, hence, aberrant attachment of the fascial coverings of the penis and spongiosum to one side, leading to torque.

Although various theories have been proposed to explain the occurrence of torsion, we believe torsion is due to abnormal attachments of the dartos fascia, Buck fascia and skin. The median raphe forms by fusion

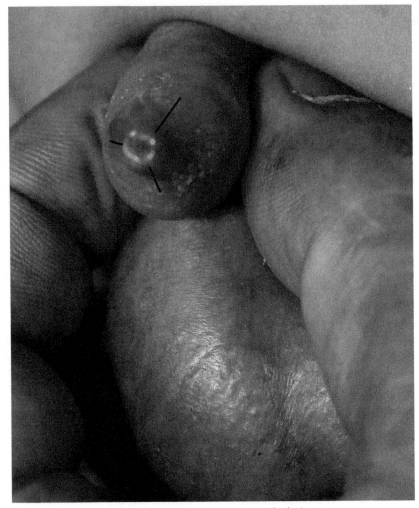

FIG. 15.4 A triple-incision preputioplasty.

of the ectodermal part of the urethral folds. Therefore during the development, if the fusion of endodermal and ectodermal components is eccentric (leading to torque), the whole penis rotates helically as a unit and the median raphe, being ventral, shifts to a direction opposite to that of the torque.[12]

The importance of recognition of torsion during circumcision lies in the fact that a simple additional manoeuvre such as penile degloving and reattaching is all that may be required for the correction of torsion. Other techniques for the repair of torsion include penile degloving with skin reattachment, dorsal dartos wrap rotation, pubic periosteal stitch, untwisting plication sutures and mobilization of the urethral plate and urethra (Fig. 15.6).[13]

CONCEALED PENIS

Concealed penis (CP) may be divided into three groups according to the Maizels[14] classification, which is based on the causative mechanism: buried penis, webbed penis and trapped penis.

In webbed penis, there is extra skin between the scrotal raphe and distal penis obscuring the penoscrotal angle. Trapped penis refers to a condition in which a normal penis is depressed under the skin following a surgical procedure, generally a circumcision, and looks concealed. Williams et al.[15] reported a rate of 9% CP among those applying for routine circumcision, and they performed a penoplasty rather than a circumcision in such cases.

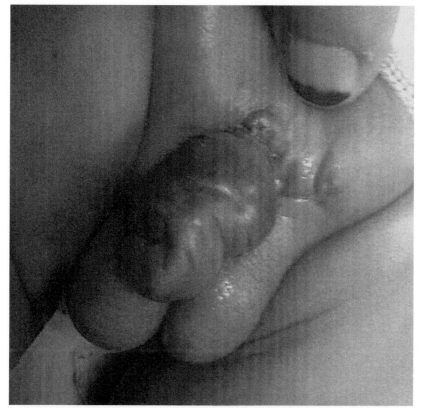

FIG. 15.5 Marked preputial lymphoedema after preputial reconstruction in hypospadias surgery.

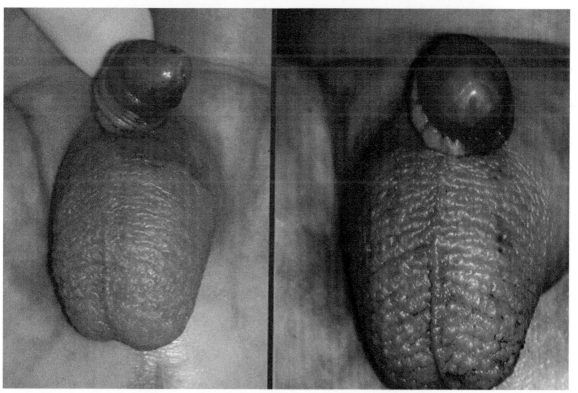

FIG. 15.6 Minor penile rotation corrected after circumcision.

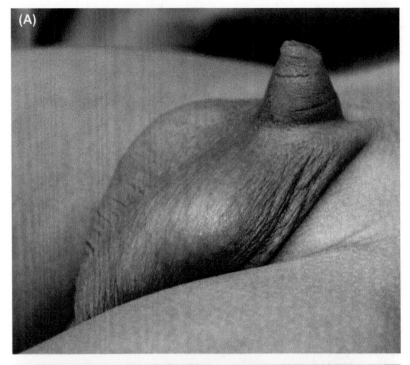

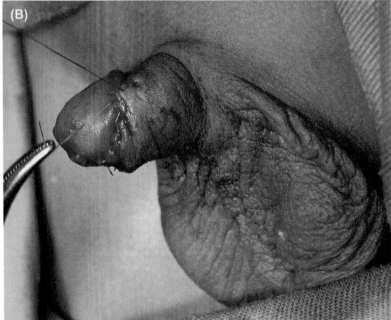

FIG. 15.7 **(A)** Concealed penis **(B)** detected and corrected during circumcision by the dissection method and partial preservation of the ventral prepuce.

The same study reported a rate of 63% CP among those applying for a circumcision revision (26% trapped penis and 37% insufficient circumcision). It is possible that one may refrain from excising sufficient prepuce to avoid more complications in a case with partial CP and insufficient circumcision may thus take place. In a baby with CP, a generous excision of the penile skin in an effort to make the penis visible leads to a crippled problem of trapped penis with almost no local penile skin surrounding the penis, requiring flaps or grafts for correction. Borsellino et al.[16] reported that a staged revision surgery was required in majority of their cases, as the penile shaft skin was also excised along with the prepuce.

Penile visibility index (PVI) calculation before circumcision might help predict the cosmetic outcome of circumcision, where the ratio of visible penile length (PL) to the stretched PL was calculated for each subject and recorded as PVI.[17]

Minor cases of CP can be detected and corrected during circumcision by the dissection method; if the surgeon has enough awareness about the surgical anatomic variation, this could be achieved through proper dissection of the tethering defective fascia and preserving the ventral aspect of the prepuce to cover the undersurface of the freed penis (Fig. 15.7).

REFERENCES

1. Cuckow PM, Cao K. Meeting the challenges of reconstructive urology — where are we now? *J Pediatr Surg*. 2018. https://doi.org/10.1016/j.jpedsurg.2018.10.070.
2. Tang SH, Kamat D, Santucci RA. Modern management of adult-acquired buried penis. *Urology*. 2008;72:124—127.
3. Schreiter F, Noll F. Mesh graft urethroplasty using split thickness skin graft or foreskin. *J Urol*. 1989;142:1223—1226.
4. Schoen EJ. Uncircumcision technique for plastic reconstruction of a prepuce after circumcision (Letter). *J Urol*. 1991;146:1619.
5. Carlisle GC. The experience of foreskin restoration: a case study. *J Psychol Christ*. 2016;35(1):83—88.
6. Purpura V, Bondioli E, Cunningham EJ, et al. The development of a decellularized extracellular matrix-based biomaterial scaffold derived from human foreskin for the purpose of foreskin reconstruction in circumcised males. *J Tissue Eng*. 2018;9. https://doi.org/10.1177/204173141 8812613, 2041731418812613. Published 2018 Dec 22.
7. Dean GE, Ritchie ML, Zaontz MR. La Vega slit procedure for the treatment of phimosis. *Urology*. 2000;55:419—421.
8. Lane TM, South LM. Lateral preputioplasty for phimosis. *J R Coll Surg Edinb*. 1999;44:310—312.
9. Wåhlin N. "Triple incision plasty". A convenient procedure for preputial relief. *Scand J Urol Nephrol*. 1992;26:107—110.
10. Wayne Griffiths R, David Bigelow J, Loewen J. Foreskin Restoration 1980—2008. In: *Genital Autonomy Book*. Dordrecht Heidelberg London New York: Springer; 2010:189—198. https://doi.org/10.1007/978-90-481-9446-9 Chapter 18.
11. Castagnetti M, Bagnara V, Rigamonti W, Cimador M, Esposito C. Preputial reconstruction in hypospadias repair. *J Pediatr Urol*. 2017;13(1):102—109. https://doi.org/10.1016/j.jpurol.2016.07.018. ISSN 1477-5131.
12. Bhat A, Bhat MP, Saxena G. Correction of penile torsion by mobilization of urethral plate and urethra. *J Pediatr Urol*. 2009;5:451—457.
13. Maizels M, Zaontz M, Donovan J. Surgical correction of the buried penis: description of a classification system and a technique to correct the disorder. *J Urol*. 1986;136:268—271.
14. Fisher PC, Park JM. Penile torsion repair using dorsal dartos flap rotation. *J Urol*. 2004;109:1903—1904.
15. Williams CP, Richardson BG, Bukowski TP. Importance of identifying the inconspicuous penis: prevention of circumcision complications. *Urology*. 2000;56:140—143. https://doi.org/10.1016/S0090-4295(00)00601-4.
16. Borsellino A, Spagnoli A, Vallasciani S, Martini L, Ferro F. Surgical approach to concealed penis: technical refinements and outcome. *Urology*. 2007;69:1195—1198. https://doi.org/10.1016/j.urology.2007.01.065.
17. Akyol I, Soydan H, Kocoglu H, Ates F, Karademir K, Baykal K. A novel tool to predict the cosmetic outcome after circumcision: penile visibility index. *Int J Clin Med*. 2014;5:605—610. https://doi.org/10.4236/ijcm.2014.510082.

Index

Note: Page numbers followed by "f" indicate figures.

Printed and bound by CPI Group (UK) Ltd, Croydon, CR0 4YY

08/05/2025

01864761-0002